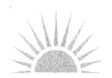

COACH'S NOTEBOOK

Games and Strategies for Lactation Education

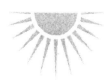

Linda J. Smith

JONES AND BARTLETT PUBLISHERS
Sudbury, Massachusetts
BOSTON   TORONTO   LONDON   SINGAPORE

World Headquarters

Jones and Bartlett Publishers
40 Tall Pine Drive
Sudbury, MA 01776
978-443-5000
info@jbpub.com
www.jbpub.com

Jones and Bartlett Publishers
Canada
6339 Ormindale Way
Mississauga, ON L5V 1J2
CANADA

Jones and Bartlett Publishers
International
Barb House, Barb Mews
London W6 7PA
UK

Jones and Bartlett's books and products are available through most bookstores and online booksellers. To contact Jones and Bartlett Publishers directly, call 800-832-0034, fax 978-443-8000, or visit our website at www.jbpub.com.

Substantial discounts on bulk quantities of Jones and Bartlett's publications are available to corporations, professional associations, and other qualified organizations. For details and specific discount information, contact the special sales department at Jones and Bartlett via the above contact information or send an email to special-sales@jbpub.com.

The authors, editor, and publisher have made every effort to provide accurate information. However, they are not responsible for errors, omissions, or for any outcomes related to the use of the contents of this book and take no responsibility for the use of the products and procedures described. Treatments and side effects described in this book may not be applicable to all people; likewise, some people may require a dose or experience a side effect that is not described herein. Drugs and medical devices are discussed that may have limited availability controlled by the Food and Drug Administration (FDA) for use only in a research study or clinical trial. Research, clinical practice, and government regulations often change the accepted standard in this field. When consideration is being given to use of any drug in the clinical setting, the health care provider or reader is responsible for determining FDA status of the drug, reading the package insert, and reviewing prescribing information for the most up-to-date recommendations on dose, precautions, and contraindications, and determining the appropriate usage for the product. This is especially important in the case of drugs that are new or seldom used.

Library of Congress Cataloging-in-Publication Data

Smith, Linda J., 1946-
  Coach's notebook : games for lactation education / Linda J. Smith.
    p. cm.
  Includes biographical references.
  ISBN 0-7637-1819-X (alk. paper)
    1. Lactation--Study and teaching--Activity programs. 2. Breast feeding--Study and teaching--Activity programs. 3. Lactation--Miscellanea. 4. Games. I. Title.

RJ216 .S557 2002
649'.33'071--dc21

                                                                        2001029658

6048

ISBN-13: 978-0-7637-1819-0
ISBN-10: 0-7637-1819-X

Production Credits
Aquisitions Editor: Penny M. Glynn
Associate Editor: Christine Tridente
Production Editor: AnnMarie Lemoine
Editorial Assistant: Thomas R. Prindle
Manufacturing Buyer: Amy Duddridge
Cover Design: Anne Spencer
Design and Composition: Pete Lippincott, D&G Limited, LLC
Printing and Binding: Courier Companies, Inc.

Printed in the United States of America
11 10 09 08 07   10 9 8 7 6 5

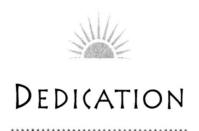

DEDICATION

*To my parents, Dorothy and Fred Dahlstrom, who made
games and sports priorities in their lives, and therefore, in mine.
They taught me good sportsmanship and the importance
of teamwork by their example.*

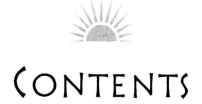

CONTENTS

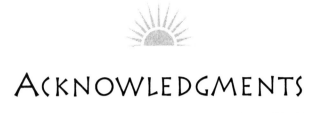

Acknowledgments

Thanks to my first swimming teacher, Ed Liebinger; my gifted swim coach, Florence Klahn; and my seventh grade homeroom and gym teacher, Florence Setter. Each of them profoundly influenced my life, encouraging my love of movement and my interest in education as a profession.

Thanks to the many talented and skilled educators who have shared their games and ideas with me, directly or indirectly, whether related to breastfeeding or other subjects. Your skill with the process of education transcends audiences and content.

A special thanks to my cheerleaders at Jones & Bartlett: Editor Penny Glynn, Associate Editor Christine Tridente, and to AnnMarie Lemoine for coaching me during the production process.

And, finally, I want to express my gratitude to the students and colleagues who have tolerated the early rough versions of these games, endured the games that "flopped," and helped me celebrate the deeper understanding and knowledge achieved through these activities.

INTRODUCTION TO COACH'S NOTEBOOK: GAMES FOR LACTATION EDUCATION

This book contains a wide variety of games and activities for teaching breastfeeding and human lactation. In writing this book, I assumed that the reader has an in-depth knowledge of breastfeeding and human lactation. All the games have been tried, tested, and refined by me and sometimes by other educators. Each activity lists the goal for the game, the ideal audience(s), the amount of time it takes to play, and specific instructions. Some of the games are very quick to implement and require little or no equipment or preparation; others are lengthy activities requiring extensive setup. Many activities are suitable for all audiences; others are more geared toward training health professionals. I have used sports analogies extensively, because breastfeeding is essentially a kinesthetic activity. The cognitive aspects of physical activities such as breastfeeding or helping mothers and babies breastfeed, playing a musical instrument, typing on a keyboard, or playing a sport are easier to learn if the teacher applies adult learning principles and interactive strategies. Combining kinesthetic, visual, and auditory learning modes nearly always results in a deeper understanding of the subject matter than any one or two learning modes used separately.

Chapter 1, "Coach's Rule Book for Using Games in Breastfeeding/Lactation Education," is an introduction to using games and interactive activities and contains recommendations for using audio-visual equipment, tips on teaching, and other helpful suggestions for the process of teaching.

Chapter 2, "Warm-ups and Stretches," is a collection of icebreakers and introductory activities suitable for opening a class or an individual course session.

Chapter 3, "On the Deck, or in the Pool?" contains games for making the decision to breastfeed and exploring the advantages of breastfeeding—or the consequences of *not* breastfeeding. These games are frequently used in parenting classes and presentations to the general public.

Chapter 4, "Drills and Lead-ups," has games for presenting specific topics or concepts in depth. A *drill* is designed to refine and polish a specific skill or aspect of an activity. A *lead-up* game explores elements of a larger game and fine-tunes specific skills or knowledge areas that will be used in the broader context of lactation management or breastfeeding care. I developed and refined some of these lead-ups throughout eight years of teaching a comprehensive lactation management course.

Chapter 5, "Secrets of the Pros," is a selection of neat and nifty ideas from master teachers from around the world. Have fun with these; they convey the uniqueness of breastfeeding in creative and effective ways.

I hope you and your audiences enjoy using these games as much as I have enjoyed developing, collecting, and compiling them.

—Coach Linda J. Smith

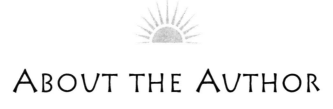

ABOUT THE AUTHOR

"Coach" Linda J. Smith develops and presents lectures, courses, and educational materials about breastfeeding management through Bright Future Lactation Resource Centre. Linda has presented lactation management/exam preparation courses to more than 1,000 people from the United States, Canada, and other countries. She is also the author of *Comprehensive Lactation Consultant Exam Review*. Her "Score Sheet for Evaluating Breastfeeding Educational Materials" was published in the *Journal of Human Lactation* in December, 1995.

Linda keeps in touch with mothers and babies as a lactation consultant in private practice in Dayton, Ohio. She helped form the International Board of Lactation Consultant Examiners and the International Lactation Consultant Association (ILCA). Linda serves on ILCA's Professional Education Council and the United States Breastfeeding Committee and is ILCA's representative to the Coalition for Improving Maternity Services (CIMS). Linda taught childbirth education classes for more than 20 years in several cities and hospitals and maintains her certification as a Lamaze Certified Childbirth Educator.

The "Coach" title comes from Linda's undergraduate degree in physical education from the State University of New York at Cortland. She has been a popular and effective teacher of diverse subjects to adults and children for more than 30 years. Her audiences range from preschool children learning tumbling to medical residents taking Basic Life Support at Wright State University School of Medicine. Her teaching venues range from coaching high school swim teams to being the keynote speaker at international lactation conferences. Linda still swims with a U.S.S. Masters team at an absurdly early hour several days a week.

1

COACH'S RULE BOOK

Using Games in
Breastfeeding and
Lactation Education

Avoiding Memories of Second Grade: Using Principles of Adult Education

Research into the principles of adult learning is transforming the entire field of education. Many adults have suffered through the rigid, dogmatic, and even punitive tactics of classroom teachers during their early educational experiences, which resulted in a fear of learning. These early fears related to the learning process can block acquisition of new ideas and facts. In contrast to old methods, effective lifelong learning is based on the following core principles:

- Continuous—learn something new almost daily.

- Purposeful—activity must make sense to the learner.

- Involves several senses—kinesthetic, visual, and auditory.

- Appropriate for the situation.

- Stimulating and interesting to the adult learners.

- Adult learners need motivation; clear and accurate demonstrations; sufficient space (both figuratively and literally); comfortable pacing and sufficient breaks; and plenty of positive feedback.

Why use games?

- Mainly because they are fun!

- Games use both sides of your brain, the spatial and verbal parts in the right and left hemispheres, and all three learning modalities—verbal, visual, and kinesthetic.

- Games trigger and foster active learning, which is far more fun and more interesting than passive learning.

- The end results are better. Concepts are usually more deeply understood and retained for a longer period of time.

- Games can help students get past unseen and sometimes unacknowledged prejudices, unhelpful beliefs, and their lack of knowledge with less threat.

The pain of using games:

* Games can take more time than lecturing.

* Games preparation can be time-consuming and tedious. If you hate arts and crafts, you may be tempted to avoid taking the time to make the necessary props for the games.

* Some theatrics are involved. Be prepared to act the part of coach, stage director, or even ringmaster.

* Some adult learners absolutely hate games, or at least think they do.

* Confessions of a sneaky teacher: Do not announce the game—just start playing it.

* Sometimes games flop. Oh well. Pick yourself up, dust yourself off, and try to salvage the point you are trying to make. Be honest—ask the audience what didn't work about the game. Was it the game format, or the information that caused problems for them?

Putting the Rabbit in the Hat: Making and Using Props

Using props and other equipment is an integral part of effective breastfeeding and lactation education. Learning is enhanced when multiple sensory modes are used. Just as you carefully prepare the content of a breastfeeding class, also pay attention to how the objects that present the content are chosen or prepared.

Dolls

Dolls are almost as good as real babies for kinesthetic teaching of positioning and latch techniques. In a way, they are better because they don't move, cry, or get overstressed. Dolls also help mothers to visualize and imagine life "after" childbirth.

It's best to always model appropriate behavior toward babies by handling dolls as you would handle a real baby. Keep dolls clean, in good repair, and dressed nicely in gender-neutral outfits. In addition, alternate between using a boy's name and a girl's name for the doll on different days and have doll(s) dressed in different outfits. Be gentle and respectful when handling dolls, especially when setting up or cleaning up the classroom.

Have students (health professionals or parents) practice positioning dolls in many of the following positions:

* Cradle (Madonna)

* Cross-cradle (cross-chest)

* Underarm (clutch, "football")

* Lying down

Some health professionals may not be familiar with the nuances of the previous breastfeeding positions. Students can also practice using tie-on soft carriers, slings, and other devices with dolls.

Weighted dolls are more expensive and sometimes are more realistic. Also be aware of skin tone, eye color, and hairstyle. Strive for a variety that approximates the characteristics of a typical audience.

Breast Models

Please do not make jokes about breast models. They are not "stuffed boobs."

Some believe that symbolically dismembering the female body, especially the reproductive organs, carries powerful negative messages about mind-body separation. Some cloth models have peel-off "skin," which shows the internal structures. Consider sewing the "skin" in place to reduce the dismembering aspect. In fact, I draw the internal structures on one surface section of the model so I can hold it either showing or hiding the drawings.

Breast models should be kept clean and in good repair and handled with respect. The skin tones of the models should vary to represent a variety of mothers.

Some commercially made breast models may also have built-in lumps for teaching breast self-examination. Whether models are handmade or purchased, make sure that there are sufficient models for all uses. I personally like the models from *Childbirth Graphics*.

Demonstrating on one's own breast, even over clothing, is controversial. Judicious use of self-modeling, such as holding a doll correctly at your own breast, is usually helpful.

Balloons

Purchase helium-quality balloons, which are resistant to breakage. The color of the balloons may matter to some audiences. Note that light colors show lipstick (used in the positioning game) better than dark colors.

Gadgets

Gadgets include breast pumps, feeding devices, and other equipment. It works best to present general information about equipment use first, before showing the specific devices. Equipment features can change rapidly, and availability may vary. There is no single *perfect* device for managing all lactation problems. Be sure to provide enough sample devices so students can handle and examine them thoroughly.

For testing breast pumps, provide plenty of extension cords and batteries and either a pressure gauge and/or sturdy balloons for demonstrating pump action. Do not ask or allow students to apply pumps or other devices to their own bodies. Always thoroughly clean all samples between demonstrations.

Game Props and Supplies

Practice using all game props before the class starts. Make sure that all parts for the game(s) are available, clean, and in good repair.

I laminate all my paper/card stock props to keep them in good condition. Store all game ("cue") cards in a zipper pouch or storage container. Remember to ask the audience to return them after use.

To make *cue cards*, use computer software to print onto white label stock, then stick the labels on blank index cards. Set the computer to print with a larger font for greater readability. Using labels to make cue cards is much faster and is usually more readable than printing directly onto card stock, which then must be trimmed into smaller pieces.

Take a lesson from marketing professionals: color sells. Brightly colored index cards or card stock generates more audience enthusiasm than plain white stock. However, be aware that some colors will pose a problem for people with visual discrimination differences. Red paper with black text is virtually unreadable by those with red-green color blindness. Text printed on patterned paper is problematic for those with visual figure-ground discrimination deficits.

Prizes are popular incentives to get students to play games. I use postcards with a breast-feeding theme, buttons, pencils, pens, or other trinkets, which I make myself or purchase from reputable sources such as La Leche League. Be aware that these items are a form of advertising. Do not use anything you receive as a gift, because that action puts you in the position of being an unpaid salesperson for a third party. If you are giving the audience a balloon, piece of candy, or another object, plan on bringing 10 percent more than you think you will need.

Specific hints on making, buying, and/or using game props and supplies are provided later with their relevant games.

Costumes and Other Gag Items

Silly hats, bells or whistles, oversized lab coats, and so on can spice up a presentation. A lecture or class without humor can make for a dry, boring presentation. However, using too much humor turns the presentation into entertainment, increasing the risk that the educational message will get lost. Be very aware of your audience, your topic, and your own lecture and teaching style before using gag items and costumes!

For example, my favorite "costume" is my bright pink ball cap with "coach" embroidered on the front. I make a show of putting on the pink hat when I'm voicing my personal or professional opinion on a topic, explaining that when the hat is off, the material that I'm presenting is well-referenced or evidence-based information. This strategy also reduces the number of evaluations which claim that, "the speaker is opinionated," about controversial topics or new information.

Murphy's Law[1] Is Alive and Well: Projection Devices and Other Equipment

Projection devices are an integral and important aspect of effective teaching because people will remember more if they can *see* your message as well as *hear* it.

The bad news is that all mechanical devices are evil, and will fail at the worst possible moment. This principle is as reliable as the law of gravity.

As a teacher, *always* have an alternate plan for presenting the information. That is what is so great about some of the games presented later—no equipment is needed!

* Focus the darn projector(s) early and often.

* Keep slides and overheads simple and easy to read. For more information on designing good visuals, refer to a book on presentation techniques such as *PowerPoint for Dummies* for tips.

* Set up and test all equipment before class. Have extra bulbs for the projector(s) on hand in case one fails and know how to replace them.

* Bring blank overheads, markers, a laser pointer with fresh batteries, and any other necessary supplies. Create a toolbox for storage of these supplies during ongoing classes.

Hauling Plastic: Overhead Transparencies

Using overhead transparencies in your classroom means the room can be kept brighter, which makes it easier for students to take notes and to stay awake and alert. Overhead projectors are easy to operate, are readily available, and are also fairly reliable.

Furthermore, overhead transparencies are also easy to make using a special marker and a plain paper copier or computer printer, and are relatively inexpensive—less than one dollar per page. For easy storage and handling, insert the transparencies into a clear (not semi-clear) page protector in a three-ring binder or tape them into cardboard frames. Lightweight page protectors are less sturdy than heavyweight, but they are lighter to lug around. Organize and number all transparencies in sequence for a given lecture. During your overhead presentation, have a table nearby to hold any unused frames and your binder.

---

[1] "If anything can go wrong, it will." There really was a Murphy. In the early days of the U.S. space program, a rocket sled was used to test the affects of sudden acceleration and deceleration. Air Force Capt. John Murphy was responsible for attaching biomedical sensors/monitors to the first human volunteer, an Air Force major who was also a physician. The sensor leads could be attached in two ways—the right way, and the wrong way. Finally, the experiment was run. The sled with the volunteer securely strapped in went screaming down the rails until the water brakes brought it to a rapid stop. The scientists eagerly examined the test instruments and found—nothing. You guessed it—all the leads had been attached backward. Capt. Murphy bravely wrote up the results, and his report found its way into our language as "Murphy's Law."

Slides—Their Pros and Cons

"There are eight ways to put slides in trays, and seven of them are wrong," says Kay Hoover, MEd, IBCLC. When the slides are in the tray correctly, label the upper right corner of each tray with a colored dot or by some other method to ensure the slides are oriented correctly in the tray. Run through the tray completely before going "live."

Make it a habit to number all the lecture slides for those times when you accidentally forget to lock the ring and the slides get dumped all over the floor.

Avoid high-density (140 slot) trays and cardboard-mounted slides because they are more likely to jam during use. (Plastic-mounted slides jam less.) Label the slides using a fine-tip, waterproof Sharpie™ marker or with Avery™ permanent labels. Keep a small metal nail file handy for rescuing stuck slides.

Seasoned instructors never, *ever* take their original slides on the road or loan them out. Instead, make duplicates of the slides, and leave the originals at home. A slight reduction in the quality of a duplicate is easier to accept than losing a unique, original slide.

Avoid presenting slides immediately after lunch or late in the afternoon, unless you want to risk putting your audience to sleep. When you use slides, the room must be darkened, which invites sleep. My personal preference is to reserve slides for showing clinical pictures because the quality of visual resolution of a 35mm slide is better than the resolution of an overhead transparency.

Video Tapes and Audio Tapes

Videos are the best way to show positioning at breast and suck patterns, and are fabulous for showing new clinical ideas. Once an audience has seen a tiny premature baby resting peacefully on its mother's chest in *Kangaroo Care*, birth in the squatting position, or a baby crawling to the breast immediately post birth, the arguments against these and other new evidence-based practices rapidly diminish.

Although videotape technology is fairly reliable, it is not foolproof. Just as with slides, never take your original tapes on the road.

A major drawback of television monitors is their small size. Depending on the size of the room, several linked monitors may be needed so everyone can view the image clearly. Note that monitors are often expensive to rent. Although wide-screen televisions and projection televisions provide larger images, they are indeed even more expensive to rent than regular monitors.

Computer-Driven Projectors

Computer-driven projectors enable you to show animations created with presentation software programs as well as videos and a wide variety of still images. A projector with at least 1000 lumens is needed for most meeting rooms having ordinary dimmed light, and may also be very expensive to buy or rent.

I really like using presentation software such as PowerPoint™ because of its ease of use and flexible options. Prepare your computer-driven presentation on at least two different media—your own laptop, a universally formatted CD-ROM, and/or a floppy disk. If you are using rented equipment, make sure the installed software supports your presentation and test it well in advance.

Microphones

Microphones are wonderful voice-savers. As an instructor, also learn how to project your voice effectively into a large room if the mike fails. Position the mike a few inches away from your mouth to prevent "popping" sounds when you pronounce certain consonants. Adjust the volume setting carefully before the session and again early in the session.

Podiums

Podiums create the effect of stiffer, formal presentations. If that is your goal, then use a podium. If you want more audience interaction or a warmer, friendlier approach, use a table to hold your equipment or props and walk around the front of the room instead.

Dress the Part

Audiences expect the speaker/teacher to look like an expert on the subject matter. Attire that is too casual can weaken credibility. Clothing should be chosen with careful consideration given to the expectations of the audience, the formality of the event, local dress styles, and your personal taste and budget. I personally always wear comfortable low-heeled shoes.

Language

Watch your language. Do not apologize, curse, or use sarcasm. Always speak clearly and a little slower than normal conversation, and avoid the temptation to rush through your lecture. Never attack other professions or professionals.

Send in the Clowns: Working with Live Humans

The comments and actions of real mothers and babies in a classroom setting is as delightful as it is unpredictable. Real nursing mothers with their babies are ideal teaching tools for all breast-feeding classes. Breastfeeding classes ideally include nursing babies of several ages including toddlers. Organizations such as a local La Leche League or Nursing Mothers may be willing to provide names. Some may argue that the sight of a nursing toddler might offend audience members. I really like to have older nursing babies in class, as well as young babies, because breastfeeding for two years or more is an essential element of the Innocenti Declaration.

Babies will usually not perform on cue. However, if the mothers and babies are available for an hour or more, at least one breastfeeding session is likely to happen. Furthermore, simply watching the mother-baby interactions is also valuable learning.

Ask the nursing mothers to talk to the group, and invite the group to directly pose questions to them. To minimize surprises, interview and prepare the mothers before class.

Occasionally a mother will give a "wrong" answer, such as "Johnny loves his pacifier" or "I think scheduled feeds are great." After the mother leaves, the instructor needs to allow sufficient time for some serious damage control.

Guest Speakers

Guest speakers break up the monotony of a single speaker. However, carefully consider the logistics and expense before inviting a guest lecturer. Surprise information (or misinformation) from a guest lecturer can be most unpleasant, and disrupt your class unless you invite the speaker repeatedly and negotiate what is going to be said. Because the guest has not heard the classroom discussions leading up to the presentation, the primary instructor needs to be prepared to provide clarification or continuity.

Role-Playing

Role-playing is generally effective and fun, but it can also backfire with dull students or those who bring their own agendas. The instructor must always be prepared with another way of covering the same material.

Disruptive Students

Disruptive students can rattle the best of teachers. Make every effort to regain control of the situation without humiliating the disruptive person. Virtually all experienced teachers, regardless of the subject matter they present, have tangled with an occasional "student from hell." A discussion of this issue with other veteran teachers will help you to develop some reliable strategies that suit your own particular teaching style and situation.

The Good, the Bad, and the Ugly: Rooms for Group Teaching

Try to avoid classroom style seating—parallel rows of chairs facing forward with the teacher positioned at the front of the room. This seating style is the least effective arrangement for learning. The following arrangements are more effective:

* Round tables are good for discussions, but the room quickly gets noisy. Large tables can be barriers to effective group work.

* A circle of chairs fosters discussion. There should be a pathway for new people to enter and others to leave the circle.

* Some games require a large open work space using empty tables, blank walls, or open floor spaces.

Allow about 35 square feet of space per person. Cramped rooms create tension; too-large rooms tend to squelch discussion.

The temperature in large buildings always varies, sometimes with annoying swings from hot to cold. Find out how to adjust your room's thermostat from the engineering staff of the building, and warn students to dress in layers.

The lighting in a large room is rarely optimal for all teaching exercises. Take the time to find out how to adjust the lighting, draperies, and so on, before the session starts, and have an assistant ready to adjust lighting as needed.

For safety reasons, be sure to tape down all cords to prevent tripping. I always bring a roll of duct tape or gaffer's tape for taping down cords.

After You Say Hello: Structuring a Lecture, Class, and Presentation

You will never be able to teach everything the students need to know. That's okay—they are only going to remember 10–50 percent of your presentation anyway.

Start and end on time. Period. Do not wait for stragglers; this just encourages tardiness. One way to get people into the room is have those already present in the room laugh uproariously or applaud enthusiastically on cue. The stragglers will rush in to see what they are missing.

Plan To Use 90 Percent

When scheduling the content of a learning session, plan to use only about 90 percent of the allotted time. Most new teachers run out of time and end up rushing through the best material that they have left for last. If all goes smoothly and if you happen to finish early, few people mind leaving early!

Ten percent of the presentation's allotted time should be for an introduction—tell them what you are going to say. Five percent of the time should be allotted for a summary—review what you have said. Then, you should divide the rest of the material into about three sections. Each section can have about three subtopics. Allow about a third of the allotted time for each topic.

When planning the content, always teach *survival* messages before *nice to know* messages. Survival messages are

* **Milk supply: How to make milk.** *Not enough milk* is the primary reason for breast-feeding failure. Making milk is the easiest and most reliable part of breastfeeding. Include what does not matter—mom's diet or fluid intake—and what does matter—frequent and thorough milk removal. Spend a lot of time thoroughly explaining the role of adequate milk transfer and milk removal from the breast to increase and maintain supply. Use current references in the explanation.

* **Comfort: How to breastfeed comfortably.** *Pain* is the second most common cause of breastfeeding failure. All pain during breastfeeding should be immediately investigated. Teach students excellent positioning and latch-on techniques (preferably using dolls) with rationales for each motion and position, and encourage mothers to get help quickly if breastfeeding is not comfortable right from the start.

* **Problems have solutions.** Do not include all the strategies for managing problems, because if the previous two survival messages are thoroughly understood, problems are rare. Just the concept that *problems can be solved* is enough of a realization at first. Always provide detailed information on getting help.

After you've taught how to breastfeed, you can include other information such as

* Motivational messages—the superiority of human milk (or, better still, the risks or drawbacks of manufactured milks)

* Milk collection and storage

* Practices that promote long-term breastfeeding (over two years)

* Policies and support from prestigious health authorities, such as the American Academy of Pediatrics (AAP) and the World Health Organization (WHO)

* Don't dwell on "benefits of breastfeeding" for the following reasons:

    - If a mother cannot produce enough milk or the process hurts her, it doesn't matter how wonderful her milk is.

    - The phrase "benefits of breastfeeding" establishes artificial feeding as the norm. Think differently—"increasing breastfeeding to 75 percent" means "reducing artificial feeding to 25 percent."

Attempts to increase motivation rarely work. Either someone *is* or *is not* motivated. Spend most of your time on the *how-to* part. Introduce the most important skills early in your class, and repeat them at the end. Teach what *to do* as well as what *not* to do.

Breastfeeding is a physical skill requiring 10–15 percent instruction and 85–90 percent practice. Babies and mothers learn to breastfeed by breastfeeding. That is to say you cannot learn to play a piano by listening to music, and if you want to make the swim team, you have to get wet.

Hanging out with the right crowd also helps. Surround yourself with like-minded people—this applies to mothers *and* professionals!

Always Choose Teams without Leaving People Out

Dividing into smaller groups breaks up cliques and puts learners slightly off-balance, which usually opens participants to new information. Here are some nonjudgmental strategies to divide a large audience into small groups:

* **By birthdays.** There are 12 months—if you need four groups, have those who were born in January, February, and March form one group, and so on. Adjust the number of months per group depending on the number of groups you need. Group size may be uneven. For just two groups, use even- or odd-numbered birthdays.

* **By count-off.** If you need four groups, go around the room with each person saying a number from one through four. All the ones will form one group, and so forth. Adjust your number range according to how many groups are needed.

* **By clothing colors.** Pick the number of colors for the number of groups you need. Announce "Everyone wearing something red form one group." Repeat until all groups are formed. If someone is not wearing any of the chosen colors, move that person into one of the smallest groups. Sometimes this method results in unequal group sizes.

* **By pre-assigned groups.** Distribute colored stick-on dots or stickers to students as they enter the room. The number of sticker colors or designs corresponds to the number of groups needed. When you want the groups to form, announce "All those with green stickers (or a snowman stamp on their packet, for example) form one group." Repeat until all groups are formed.

* **By announcing "Everyone find a partner" or "Form groups of three" and so on.** This method can be awkward for some and can result in some people remaining in their seats. A drawback is that some participants tend to work with a friend, which may not enhance learning. The worst drawback is that someone will be the *odd one out* or left standing alone. Nobody likes to be the last person chosen.

Post-Mortems and Wrap-ups: Formal and Informal Evaluations

"Although tests are optional [for classes and courses], evaluations are not," writes Helen Armstrong, MAT, IBCLC; UNICEF trainer and consultant. Feedback from students is essential.

Ask students directly for feedback during breaks, lunches, and other contact points. Also, you can have other staff members or instructors listen for comments about the class.

Subjective evaluations address the students' feelings and emotions about the class or about the material presented. Here are some examples:

* What surprised you most about today's session?

* What is the most outrageous thing you have heard about breastfeeding?

    – My biggest Ah-HAH! today was. . .

    – I wish I had known that. . .

    – I would have learned the material better if. . .

To get responses that tell you what you want to know, write your evaluation questions carefully and review them periodically.

Objective evaluations are usually required if you are obtaining a continuing education credit, although they may not provide adequate feedback. The best source I have found is *Preparing Instructional Objectives* by Robert Mager, PhD.

Read all the evaluations you receive. A word of warning: *don't think about elephants.* In other words, resist the temptation to obsess on the inevitable (and hopefully few) negative comments that you read. When a student is angry enough to write a nasty evaluation, your information probably had a profound impact on that person, which may open that person's mind to new ideas.

Do look for substantive and repeating ideas and themes in both negative and positive evaluations, such as content areas that could be presented differently, any environmental factors that can be changed, or a teaching method in need of work.

Take the time to write your own evaluation for every class and course you teach. I prepare formal evaluation forms for each day's material and each course as a whole, and make a point to complete them. I either make the change in the material immediately after a class, or review all my notes and make changes as I'm preparing for the next time the course is given.

Review *everything* you teach at least once a year. The half-life of breastfeeding information seems to be about five years, and new research often changes our views and practices.

And finally,

"Always leave 'em wanting more."

—P. T. Barnum.

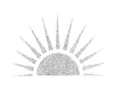

THE
GAMES

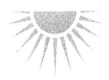

2

WARM-UPS AND STRETCHES

Introductions and Icebreakers

FIND SOMEONE WHO

GOAL

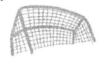

Introduce core breastfeeding concepts and behaviors by exploring personal experiences of the group. Promote group cohesiveness and camaraderie.

BEST AUDIENCE

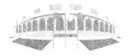

20 or more adult women. The game can be modified for mixed gender groups, teenagers, or other groups.

TIME REQUIRED

10–15 minutes

HOW TO PLAY

Distribute one form for each person in the group and have them get out a pen or pencil.

Find a person who fits each of the 20 items from the list on your paper. Ask one person to initial or sign your paper on the relevant line. You can sign as many *other* lists as you wish, but you can sign only *one* line per paper. You may *not* sign your own list. The first person to get all their lines filled in wins. (Alternate: The game ends when everyone has their list completely signed.)

Tips on playing:

- Include the instructor(s) in the group.

- If there are fewer than 20 people in the group, allow each person to sign on more than one line.

- More than half of the statements are related to breastfeeding. Do not remove any items related to breastfeeding—each covers a different aspect of breastfeeding. You can substitute other *breastfeeding* statements such as the following:

  - Works at a Baby Friendly™ hospital

  - Wrote a book, article, or publication about breastfeeding

  – Took a breastfeeding or lactation management course that was at least three days long

  – Owns at least five professional breastfeeding books

  – Owns a doll that either gives birth or breastfeeds her "baby"

  – Subscribes online to Lactnet or to another breastfeeding list on the Internet

  – Watched a sibling being breastfed

* The addition of more items can sometimes slow down the game.

* Other possible (replacement) items *not related to breastfeeding*:

  – Has lived outside this country, this state or province

  – Knows how to sail a boat, drive a tractor, or ride a motorcycle

  – Has played a competitive sport

  – Hates gardening/yard work

  – Does not own a television

  – Does not like chocolate

  – Is really good at driving in the snow

  – Has been through a flood, tornado, or hurricane

  – Owns a pair of green shoes, bell-bottom pants, or string of love beads

FIND SOMEONE WHO. . .

Find someone who fulfills each of the following criteria and have each person initial the lines which pertain to him or her. Get a *different* person for each line.

1. Breastfed a premature baby or helped a mother who did _____

2. Sleeps with a dog or cat on their bed _____

3. Overcame nipple pain and continued to breastfeed _____

4. Has three or more children _____

5. Breastfed twins or triplets or helped someone who did _____

6. Breastfed all her children _____

7. Is not married _____

8. Has only female children _____

9. Used an electric breast pump _____

10. Exercises at least three times a week _____

11. Never gave her baby formula, not even once _____

12. Breastfed longer than one year _____

13. Can play a musical instrument _____

14. Has only male children _____

15. Received help from La Leche League _____

16. Taught a prenatal breastfeeding class _____

17. Never breastfed a baby _____

18. Follows the *family bed* concept
    (practiced co-sleeping with their baby or child) _____

19. Is a grandmother _____

20. Never, ever had a traffic ticket _____

WHO'S GLAD YOU'RE BREASTFEEDING?

GOAL

To look at the *advantages* of breastfeeding for others beside the baby and mother.

BEST AUDIENCE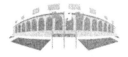

Any group of more than 10 people

TIME REQUIRED

10–15 minutes

HOW TO PLAY

There are two ways to play this game. For the fill-in-the-blank method, the group leader supplies a list of 10–20 people who are glad that you are breastfeeding. For the freewheeling method, start the game with three to four examples, and then solicit contributions from the group. Be prepared with references to support each item.

Format: <Person/Profession> is glad that I am breastfeeding because <advantage for that person>.

Example: <My pediatrician> is glad that I am breastfeeding because <my baby is healthier, growing well, and is happy and content>.

Who is glad	Why he or she is glad (These are only suggested responses—there are more!)
The garbage collector	Breastfed babies fill fewer diapers, and the used diapers smell better besides.
Our accountant	Breastfeeding saves the family (or company) money.
Mensa (club for people with high I.Q.)	Breastfed babies are smarter, and they can join *Mensa* later on.
My gynecologist	Faster recovery from birth; aids family planning; less cancer.
The ear, nose, and throat doctor	Baby has far fewer ENT infections.
My husband	Cost savings; healthier; wife gets up at night.
The flight attendant on a plane	Baby is quieter—mother can nurse during takeoff and landing.
Weight Watchers leader	Lose weight faster post birth.
My boss/employer	Employee is at work more, and loses fewer work days at home with a sick child.
Our family dentist	Strong jaw muscles.
The school athletic coach	Better eye-hand coordination and motor development.

continues

continued

Who is glad	Why he or she is glad
The dermatologist	Fewer skin blemishes—especially those caused by allergy.
The allergist	Fewer allergies.
The washing machine repairman	Human milk washes out of clothing and diapers easily without staining, reducing wear and tear on the appliances.
The government	Supports national health goals.
The formula company	Partial breastfeeding sells more formula which is advertised as the *next best* thing to mother's own milk.
The social service agency	Better bonding.
Baby shoe manufacturers	Breastfed babies walk sooner.
Our orthodontist	Less orthodontia is needed.
I'm glad	Wonderful bond; convenient; fun.

Source: *Lactation Consultant in Private Practice* conference, Philadelphia, PA.

SECRET SUCCESS

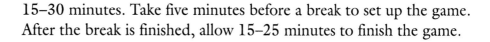

GOAL

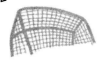

To bolster or reinforce the self-esteem of students.

BEST AUDIENCE

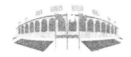

Any group that meets more than two or three times. The game is ideally used midway through a multisession course or class series.

TIME REQUIRED

15–30 minutes. Take five minutes before a break to set up the game. After the break is finished, allow 15–25 minutes to finish the game.

HOW TO PLAY

Distribute small pieces of paper to each person in the group. Before dismissing the group for a break, ask each person to briefly write down (on the paper) a personal victory that he or she accomplished in the past few months to a year. It should *not* be something that a spouse or child accomplished, or something that happened by pure luck, but a personal accomplishment that makes the person feel proud. Then, gather up and fold the papers, put them into a container, and mix them around.

After the break, each returning person takes a paper and reads it privately. The game is to find the person who wrote the paper you selected, and to be found by the person who has the paper written by you.

When everyone has been found, every paper is read to the group and all the victories are celebrated.

"Did You Know" Table Tents

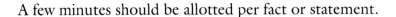

GOAL

Present the facts about breastfeeding, breastfeeding advocacy, or other relevant discussion topics during a meal or in waiting areas.

BEST AUDIENCE

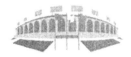

Professional workshops and conferences, or in waiting rooms areas (for example, in clinics).

TIME REQUIRED

A few minutes should be allotted per fact or statement.

HOW TO PLAY

Prepare a set of *Did You Know* table tents (folded pieces of card stock that sit like tents on a tabletop) or index cards. One way is to print the statements on computer-ready labels, and then stick them onto index cards. Lamination also makes the tents or cards more durable for repeated use.

The information on the tents or cards should include facts about breastfeeding, disease statistics related to infant feeding, political issues, famous women who breastfed their babies, famous people who were breastfed, and so forth.

You can make the tents/cards one-sided, self-contained pieces of information. Or, they can be designed with two parts—a brief state-ment or question on the front or outside, with a sentence or two on the back or inside. See the trivia list for statement ideas.

Place one tent/card on each table during a meal, or place one or two on a table in a waiting area. For clinic use, switch cards frequently.

BREASTFEEDING TRIVIA

GOAL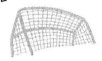

Capture an audience's attention with interesting facts about breastfeeding, breastfeeding associations, and the lactation consultant profession.

BEST AUDIENCE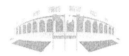

Health care professionals and lactation management students. Some individual trivia items are also suitable for parents or the general public.

TIME REQUIRED

Time required: Variable

HOW TO PLAY

Use any or all of the questions and answers for any of the following reasons:

- As icebreakers
- To recapture an audience's attention
- As an excuse to award a prize in the middle of a presentation on an otherwise dry topic
- As table tents for discussion groups
- For other purposes

These items are not listed in any particular order.

Question	Answer
Who wrote the 1981 *Petition to Alleviate Domestic Infant Formula Abuse?*	Angela Blackwell of Public Advocates, Inc., San Francisco, CA
When was the first edition of *Breastfeeding, a Guide for the Medical Profession* published?	Ruth A. Lawrence, MD, wrote this first medical textbook on breastfeeding in 1980.
What color was the cover of the first edition of the *Womanly Art of Breastfeeding?*	The first edition cover was white. The cover of the second edition was blue.
What was Karen Pryor's profession when she wrote the first edition of *Nursing Your Baby?*	Dolphin trainer/marine scientist
Who wrote *Breastfeeding in Practice?*	Elisabet Helsing
On what date was UNICEF's *Baby Friendly Hospital Initiative* announced in the USA?	March 9, 1992
Who programmed the first ILCA membership database and on what computer and software was it programmed?	Dennis L. Smith, using a Commodore 64® computer running The Consultant™ software. This software was state-of-the art for personal computers in early 1985.
Who was the first Secretary on ILCA's Board of Directors?	Linda Smith held the position from 1985–1988.
Name all the members of ILCA's founding Board of Directors.	Faith Bedford (President), Trina Vosti (Vice President), Kathy Warmbier (Treasurer), Linda Smith (Secretary), Candace Woessner (President-elect), Linda Kutner (U.S. delegate.), Lynn Stewart (Canadian delegate), Evi Adams (International delegate)

Question	Answer
What was the title of the ILCA publication that preceded the *Journal of Human Lactation*?	*Consultant's Corner.* Before this journal began, La Leche League's Lactation Consultant Department published a newsletter named "Droplets."
Name the members of the first Exam Committee for the International Board of Lactation Consultant Examiners (IBLCE).	Linda Smith, Eileen Leaphart, Sarah Danner, Jeanne Driscoll, Kathy Auerbach, JoAnne Scott, and Leon Gross (psychometrician).
Where and when was the first and only joint ILCA—La Leche League conference?	In San Diego, 1986. One day of La Leche League International's Physician's Seminar was jointly sponsored by ILCA.
What color was the cover of the first ILCA membership directory?	It was green and was published in 1985.
What year was the first ILCA conference outside of the United States?	1989 in Toronto, Ontario Canada
When was the first research article on cup-feeding published?	The first article on cup-feeding of infants was published in 1948. —Davis HV, Sears RR, Miller HC, Brodbeck AJ. Effects of cup, bottle and breastfeeding on oral activities of newborn infants. *Pediatrics* 1948; 2:549-55.
When did research show that breastfed babies walk about two months earlier than those artificially fed?	This was first reported in 1929. —Hoefer C, Hardy MC. Later development of breastfed and artificially fed infants. *J Am Med Assoc* 1929; 92:615.
How fast do a mother's breasts produce milk?	They produce 11–58 ml of milk per hour per breast, according to research by Peter Hartmann, PhD of Perth, Australia.

continues

continued

Question	Answer
What is the recommended normal vacuum pressure of a hospital-grade electric breast pump?	It is about 100–250 mm Hg, according to research by Einer Egnell.
Where, when, and by whom were the first breastfeeding clinics in the United States established?	Audrey Naylor, MD, DrPH and Ruth Wester, RN, CPNP, started the San Diego Lactation Program at University of California San Diego in 1977, which was incorporated as Wellstart International in 1985. In 1979, Chele Marmet and Ellen Shell founded the Lactation Institute in Los Angeles. Edward Cerutti, MD, and Sarah Danner, RN, CPNP, CNM opened the Lactation Clinic in Cleveland, Ohio in 1981.
Where and when was "rooming-in" first implemented in the United States?	Edith Jackson, MD implemented rooming-in at Yale University Hospital in New Haven, CT in 1952. —Barnes BF, Lethin AN, Jackson EB et al. Management of breastfeeding. *J Am Med Assoc* 1953; 151:192.
When did ILCA commit to endorsing the World Health Organization's *International Code of Marketing of Breastmilk Substitutes* (W.H.O. Code?)	It was endorsed in 1988 by a unanimous vote by the Board of Directors. Since 1988, ILCA has taken a strong stand in support of the Code.
What group was the first affiliate of ILCA?	The Michigan Association of Lactation Consultants (MALC), organized by Jan DeCoopman.
When and where was the *Innocenti Declaration* signed?	This global action plan for breastfeeding was signed on August 1, 1990, in Florence, Italy.
Where did Kangaroo Care originate?	Bogota, Columbia
Which component of cow's milk has no counterpart in human milk?	Beta lactoglobulin, which is the dominant protein in cow's milk

Question	Answer
When was the Human Milk Banking Association of North America established?	HMBANA was established in 1985, the same year that ILCA was founded.
Who first examined breastfeeding education in U.S. medical schools?	Edward Newton, MD —Newton ER. Breastfeeding/lactation and the medical school curriculum. *J Hum Lact* 1992; 8:122.
Who was the first president of La Leche League International?	Marian Thompson
Who developed the Dancer hand position?	Sarah Coulter Danner, RN, CPNP, CNM, IBCLC and Ed Cerutti, MD. Dancer comes from the first letters of their last names (Dan + Cer).
As of the year 2000, what is the highest score ever earned on the IBLCE exam?	95 percent. It was earned by a candidate from Australia in 2000.
Who was the first physician and first male to take the IBLCE exam?	Jay Gordon, MD, in 1985. Dr. Gordon is a pediatrician in California.
Where was the first IBLCE exam site outside the United States?	Melbourne, Australia in 1985
Which protective factor *increases* when human milk is frozen?	Lysozyme
The withdrawal of which hormone triggers the onset of copious milk secretion post birth?	Progesterone is withdrawn when the placenta is delivered, which triggers lactogenesis II, the onset of copious milk secretion, 30–40 hours later.
What percent of pediatric office visits in the United States during the child's first year of life are due to allergy?	One-third

continues

continued

Question	Answer
When and where was La Leche League International founded?	LLLI was founded in Chicago, Illinois, in 1956 by seven women.
Name one of the hospitals shown in the video *A Healthier Baby by Breastfeeding*.	Good Samaritan Hospital in Dayton OH or Charlotte Memorial Hospital in Charlotte, NC
When did La Leche League begin offering *Breastfeeding Seminars for Physicians*?	The Physicians' Seminars were started in 1973. Dr. Lawrence Gartner, MD was the primary driving force in developing these effective and popular seminars.
What is the average volume of milk synthesized (made) by one mother for a single baby in the first six months?	One woman's average volume of milk synthesized for one baby is about one liter per day. However, the amount can widely vary depending on the baby's needs.
How much formula would a baby have to consume to get the same amount of immune protection as in one ounce of colostrum?	This is a trick question. Formula cannot duplicate the protective factors in colostrum.
What method of family planning prevents more unplanned pregnancies than all others combined?	Breastfeeding. In addition, global clinical trials have verified the efficacy of the Lactational Amennorrhea Method (LAM).
Why were the formulas NeoMulSoy™ and Cho-Free™ taken off the market in 1980?	They lacked chloride, which is an essential nutrient for brain development. Lynn Pilot and Carol Laskin formed Formula, Inc., to investigate the risks of chloride-free formulas and other related issues.
Who said "If a mother decides to feed with formula, the reasons should be explored in case the decision was based on a misconception?"	The American Academy of Pediatrics and the American College of Obstetricians and Gynecologists, in *Guidelines for Perinatal Care*, published in 1992.

Question	Answer
How long do women's breasts continue to produce milk after the last breastfeeding?	No one knows for sure, but some research suggests milk synthesis continues for at least 42 days after the last feeding.
Name some famous women who have breastfed their babies.	Lynne Redgrave, Cybil Shepherd (twins), Princess Diana, Princess Grace of Monaco, Cathy Rigby, Katherine Ross, Natalie Wood, Jane Pauly, Joan Lunden, Mia Farrow, Linda Kelsey, Jayne Kennedy, Susan St. James, Lady MacBeth, Demi Moore, Meryl Streep, Deborah Norville, Meredith Baxter-Birney, Mariette Hartley, Olivia Newton-John, Mary (mother of Jesus), Chris Evert, Hillary Rodham Clinton, Bette Midler, Kathie Lee Gifford, Tipper Gore, Rhea Perlman, Tanya Tucker, Shelley Long, and Delores Jordan, Michael Jordan's mother
Why is colostrum yellow?	Colostrum is yellow because it contains large amounts of Beta-carotene. Beta-carotene is an antioxidant which protects the gut from many diseases. Vegetables containing Beta-carotene have high amounts of Vitamin A and have been found to reduce the risk of cancers of the digestive system in adults.
What fatty acid constitutes 55 percent of the dry weight of an infant brain?	Docosohexanoic acid (DHA). DHA is concentrated in the brain and retina. There is no DHA naturally found in infant formula. Human milk and marine oils (i.e., cod liver oil) are the best sources of this nutrient, which is important in cognitive development and visual acuity (especially for premature babies).
What is the most common ingested allergen in infants?	The most common ingested allergen in infants is cow's milk protein. An allergy to soy protein is also common.

continues

continued

Question	Answer
Why is milk white?	Milk is white because it contains large amounts of casein, the milk protein that is rich in calcium. Another milk protein is whey, which appears clear or watery. Many of the immunoglobulins and protective proteins are found in the whey portion of milk. Women's milk is about 80 percent whey and 20 percent casein, and quickly travels through a baby's digestive system. Cow's milk is about 80 percent casein, which forms big curds in the calf's stomach that are digested very slowly. Cow's milk is cloudy and chalky because it's higher in casein. Casein can be made into cheese. A trick to remember these differences: *W* stands for *Women's* milk, high in *Whey*, *Wonderful Immunoglobulins*, and makes for *Whiz*-bang smart kids. *C* stands for *Cow's* milk, high in *Casein*, *Chalky* and ideal for making *Chewy Curds* for *Calves*.
How much profit does the infant formula industry make every year?	About eight billion (U.S.) dollars
Which U.S. senator conducted hearings on infant formula marketing in 1981?	Senator Edward M. (Ted) Kennedy. These hearings and other investigations led to the development of the World Health Organization's *International Code of Marketing of Breastmilk Substitutes*, which the United States endorsed by consensus in 1994.
Where did the idea of forming ILCA (the International Lactation Consultant Association) originate?	Linda Smith and Joanne Scott were discussing the development of what became IBLCE one day in 1984, and Linda said, "We need to form a new association."

Question	Answer
How often do adults feel an urge to eat?	Every 90 minutes
Where did the *Suckle Up* bumper stickers first appear?	They first appeared in San Diego, in 1986. The print shop working on the first ILCA conference created them.
When a baby is properly nursing, what is the angle of opening of his or her jaw?	"Over 120 degrees," observes Kay Hoover.
How much does lead poisoning lower a child's I.Q. score?	Lead poisoning lowers I.Q. by about four points. Formula reduces the I.Q. of tube-fed preemies by about twice that amount. —Lucas A, Morley R, Cole TJ, et al. Breastmilk and subsequent intelligence quotient in children born preterm. *Lancet* 1992: 339; 261–64.
When was the World Alliance for Breastfeeding Advocacy (WABA) founded?	WABA was started in 1991.
Where and when was the first IBLCE exam held?	Washington, D.C. and Melbourne, Australia, in 1985. It was the first health credentialling board to test internationally.
When did the United States pass the Infant Formula Act, which regulates the composition of formulas?	The Infant Formula Act was passed in 1980. It regulates the allowable minimum levels of some nutrients in standard formulas.
Who wrote *Maternal Emotions*?	Niles Newton, PhD in 1955
When did the U.S. WIC (Supplemental Food Program for Women, Infants and Children) first designate funds for breastfeeding?	Specific funds for breastfeeding were designated in 1989, thanks to the efforts of Nancy Schweers, Minda Lazarov, Barbara Howell, and others.

continues

continued

Question	Answer
When did the U.S. pass a law prohibiting the price-fixing of infant formula used in the WIC program?	1992
Which U.S. president signed the Breastfeeding Promotion Act in 1992?	George Bush. This law supports U.S. national breastfeeding promotion activities.
According to Mitchell, what are the three most important factors associated with cot death (i.e., SIDS)?	Maternal smoking, prone sleep position, and artificial feeding. Those three factors account for 79 percent of the SIDS deaths in New Zealand in his 1991 study. —Mitchell EA, Stewart MW, Becroft DM et al. Results from the first year of the New Zealand cot death study. *NZ Med J* 104: 71–76, 1991.
How many nerve connections does the baby form in the first two years?	14,000 nerve endings are formed in the first two years. Stroking and touching fosters the growth of these nerve fibers.
Who developed a lactation curriculum for medical schools?	Wellstart International in May 1994

3

ON THE DECK, OR IN THE POOL?

Games for Exploring the
Decision to Breastfeed

COOKIE GAME[1]

GOAL

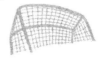

To learn emotional messages conveyed by foods and to relate them to milk composition.

BEST AUDIENCE

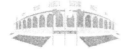

Anyone

TIME REQUIRED

One minute at the beginning of a break, then 10 minutes when the group reconvenes after the break.

HOW TO PLAY

As the group gets ready for a break, set out two plates of similar cookies—one plate of homemade cookies and one plate of an obviously cheap, commercially available type. Invite all the group members to take a cookie as they leave. When they get back, ask them which cookie they took and why they took the one they did.

Their answers will be easy to correlate to the advantages of breast milk/breastfeeding. The homemade cookies usually are taken quickly, leaving the cheap, commercially available ones. The following examples are answers that are commonly given:

- The homemade ones are made with love.

- I know what is in them—you don't know what is in the bagged ones.

Be prepared for someone to like the predictability or uniformity of the cheap cookies or worry about making others feel guilty. Use this opportunity to point out the need for an ingredient list on any manufactured product.

---

[1] **Source:** I learned this game from Suzanne Hilbers, RPT, FACCE.

Variations:

- I watch the plates. If all the homemade cookies are gone, I take away the plates. Sometimes the store-bought ones go too, but only after the good ones. I've also put the homemade ones on a nice plate or basket and the store-bought ones in their opened wrapper, which brings up the discussion of the container.

  —Kym Smythe, MEd, IBCLC; Bear, DE

- Try this game with homemade whole wheat bread and store-bought white bread.

  —Anne Cook, MS, LLL leader; Sturgis, MI

- The speaker passes out the cookies, choosing who gets which type. This is much like the baby's perspective—who ends up fed human milk, and who ends up fed formula.

  —Leslie Ward, Fort Hood, TX and Pat Young, MSN, IBCLC; Pitman, NJ

FEEDING LINE GAME[2]

....

GOAL

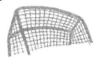

To explore the attitudes and lifestyles relating to infant feeding.

BEST AUDIENCE

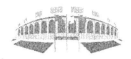

Prenatal childbirth class or generic infant-feeding class. This game can also be used as an introductory in-service for professionals.

TIME REQUIRED

15–20 minutes for under 20 participants

HOW TO PLAY

Imagine there is a line diagonally across the room, which is numbered from 0 to 10 from one end to the other. Zero represents exclusive formula feeding and 10 represents exclusive breastfeeding (directly from the breast with no pacifiers, bottles, or pumping).

On your signal, have everyone in the group stand on a number which represents how that person thinks they might approach infant feeding. The instructor asks each person why he or she chose that specific number.

Then, after a second signal, each person must move to a different number and explain that new position. *This step must be included.* Instead of going down the line, asking each person in order why he or she took that position, it works best to pick people randomly from various positions on the line, making sure that everyone who wants to respond has been given that opportunity.

---

[2] **Source**: This game is modified from a similar activity that explores the methods of pain relief for labor and birth as presented by Suzanne Hilbers, RPT, FACCE.

As the instructor, you can comment on advantages, pros/cons, and so forth, either before, during, or after this exercise. Personally, I think it works best to add your comments afterwards. Keep the discussion focused on the theme of *possibilities* to avoid dogmatic confrontations. It is also helpful to present unvoiced sides of the issue whenever possible, especially when the discussion turns to the costs and risks of artificial and mixed feedings.

When the participants change places, they should treat the change as a *walk in someone else's shoes* and mention the other/different perspective. Having each person speak about *two* positions helps individuals to understand other viewpoints. It also helps to bring forth comments which will likely be heard by the mother or professionals, enabling them to think through their responses.

EVERYBODY'S DOING IT³

GOAL

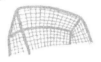

To explore some unique advantages of breastfeeding in a slightly risqué, humorous way. This game can also be used as an icebreaker.

BEST AUDIENCE

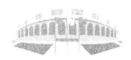

Groups of at least 10 people—parents or professionals. For smaller groups, the entire group can play as one team.

TIME REQUIRED

10–20 minutes

HOW TO PLAY

Prepare one or more sets of *Doing It* cards. Divide the group into 10 teams. Give each team one card (i.e., one statement). To illustrate the game's title, "Everybody's Doing It," either prepare a card for this statement, which treats it like the other statements, or have the entire group present this statement. Allow 5–10 minutes for teams to decide how to illustrate, act out, sing, read, or otherwise present their statement. When all teams are ready, each team will present its statement to the re-assembled group.

³ **Source:** Members of the Ithaca NY Breastfeeding Coalition wrote the statements used in the game.

THE STATEMENTS

* I can do it for an hour and not get sore.

* We love to do it in bed.

* I did it with two girls at once.

* At first my mother said I shouldn't do it, but when she watched us, she changed her mind.

* We do it at the movies.

* I can walk and do it at the same time.

* I read while I do it.

* The longer we do it, the healthier we both are.

* It's the most satisfying thing I've ever done.

* He's short, and fat, and nearly bald . . . and he's really good at it!

* Breastfeeding—Everybody's doing it!

THE GUILT GAME, OR IF ONLY I HAD KNOWN

GOAL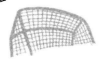

To explore negative feelings related to feeding choices such as guilt from unmet expectations; regret from making choices that seemed right at the time; sadness for not implementing a choice for lack of support, incorrect information, and so forth.

BEST AUDIENCE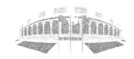

Parents having subsequent children and/or health professionals who are expected to promote and support breastfeeding regardless of their personal beliefs, decisions, or success at breastfeeding.

TIME REQUIRED

15–20 minutes

HOW TO PLAY

Begin the game by distributing research conclusions about health differences in breastfeeding, such as the FactPacks™ and/or NicePacks™ by posting them on the walls, by spreading them out on the floor (use laminated ones), or by passing them out to participants (use flashcard size). Personally, I like the on-the-floor method best. Ask the participants to then walk around or exchange the cards and find at least one statement that is new information to them. Then reconvene the group and introduce the following topic:

We all make decisions with the information we have *at that time*. Later, as new information comes to light, we often have second thoughts about those original decisions. For those of you with children: If you were having your first baby *now*, what would you do differently? For those without children, what do you see parents doing now that is different from what you were seeing a few years ago?

45

The answers to this question may include using car seats, being more gentle, brushing the children's teeth more, and so on. Point out that hindsight always reveals information which was lacking at the time an important decision was made.

Then, have the group think about the fact(s) provided on the cards they read. Ask them, "How does this research information on infant feeding make you feel?" Participants will probably answer with surprise, disbelief, some anger, sadness, guilt, defensiveness, and some pride. Let these answers lead into a discussion on grieving and guilt. The *guilt* related to breastfeeding probably comes from one of the following two sources:

- A belief that breastfeeding does not matter, and then later finding out that it *did* matter, thereby regretting the missed opportunity

  or

- Wanting to breastfeed but failing because of some problem or lack of information

The way to protect women from this guilt is twofold:

1. Provide sufficient information so women can make more informed decisions

2. Ensure that all women have access to skilled, timely help for preventing and resolving problems

Promotion only, without adequate and knowledgeable sources of support, may exacerbate the guilt associated with breastfeeding.

Conclude this game by stressing the importance of learning and teaching accurate information on the *how* of breastfeeding.

Note: These cards can also be used with first-time parents. Focus on the advantages of breastfeeding that they have never heard before, and the ideas which might make them commit more fully to breastfeeding their babies. Conclude with providing specific sources which will help with the *how* of breastfeeding.

Tip: The Breastfeeding Quiz, located later in the chapter, is one source of research-based facts which can be used in this game.

TREASURE HUNT
("BREASTFEEDING IS") GAME

GOAL

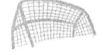

To explore the motivational themes for breastfeeding promotion.

BEST AUDIENCE

Any

TIME REQUIRED

Five minutes to prepare the room; 10–15 minutes to play the game.

HOW TO PLAY

Equipment needed: One set of 16 "Breastfeeding Is" buttons, and one set of 16 "Breastfeeding Is" cards. If possible, supply enough sets [or add new referenced statements] so that each player can find one button or card.

Before the class begins, hide the 16 "Breastfeeding Is" buttons and the corresponding 16 "Breastfeeding Is" cards around the room. Ideally, there should be one button or card for each person. When the group is assembled, announce that the group will play a Treasure Hunt for buttons and cards. The rules are that each person must only claim *one* button or card, then must stand aside for others to find the rest. Then announce, "Ready—Set—GO!"

After all buttons and cards have been found, have the card-finders and button-finders pair up according to the statements they have found. As partners, they should then discuss the teaching points with each other, and read the teaching point to the class afterwards. Finally ask, "Who learned something new?" and "Which ideas, if any, would have made a difference to *you?*"

Conclude the game with a discussion about the motivational messages for breastfeeding, including "What is in it for Mom?"

If you have sufficient resources, allow the participants to keep the items they found. Otherwise, collect the items for future use.

Breastfeeding (BF) Is. . .	Teaching Points	References
Accessible	BF ensures the baby's frequent and intimate access to Mom; importance of skin touch to development.	Winnicott, Donald W. *Babies and Their Mothers*. Reading: Addison-Wesley Publishing, 1987. Montagu, Ashley. *Touching: the Human Significance of the Skin*. New York: Harper and Row, 1971 and 1978.
Best	Global significance of BF, which is recommended for *all babies* and *all mothers*	UNICEF. *Facts for Life: A Communication Challenge*. New York: UNICEF, 1990. Institute of Medicine (Subcommittee on Nutrition During Lactation, Food and Nutrition Board). *Nutrition During Lactation*. Washington, D.C.: National Academy of Sciences, 1991.
Easy	BF is comfortable and convenient; making good quality milk is easy; help is available.	Renfrew M, Fisher C, Arms S. *The New Bestfeeding: Getting Breastfeeding Right for You*. Berkeley: Celestial Arts, 2000. La Leche League International. *The Womanly Art of Breastfeeding*. Schaumburg, IL: La Leche League International, 1997.

Breastfeeding (BF) Is. . .	Teaching Points	References
Empowering	Mother's confidence and self-esteem are strengthened and enhanced by BF.	Locklin MP, Naber SJ. Does breastfeeding empower women? Insights from a select group of educated, low-income, minority women. *Birth* 1993; 20(1): 30–35. Kitzinger, Sheila. *Breastfeeding Your Baby.* New York: Alfred A. Knopf, 1989.
Friendly	Baby Friendly™ practices that support BF are good for all mothers and babies worldwide.	World Health Organization (WHO)/UNICEF. *Protecting, Promoting and Supporting Breastfeeding: the Special Role of Maternity Services.* Geneva, Switzerland: WHO, New York: UNICEF, 1989 (includes the Baby Friendly Hospital Initiative).
Fun	Moms enjoy BF. This is also a political issue of women's rights.	Bumgarner, NJ. *Mothering Your Nursing Toddler.* Schaumburg IL: La Leche League International, 2000. Palmer, G. *The Politics of Breastfeeding.* London: Pandora Press, 1994.
Healthy	Artificial feeding has significant short and long term risks to mothers, babies, and families.	Cunningham AS, Jelliffe DB, Jelliffe EFP. Breastfeeding and health in the 1980s: a global epidemiologic review. *Journal of Pediatrics* 1991; 18(5): 659–666. Dewey KG, Heinig J, Nommsen-Rivers L. Differences in morbidity between breastfed and formula-fed infants. *Journal of Pediatrics* 1995; 126: 696–702.

continues

continued

Breastfeeding (BF) Is. . .	Teaching Points	References
Natural	BF has significant ecological impact. Industries that support artificial feeding waste resources.	Radford A. The ecological empact of bottle-feeding. *Breastfeeding Review* 1992; 5: 204–208. Frank JW, et al. Breastfeeding in a polluted world: uncertain risks, clear benefits. *Canadian Medical Association Journal* 1993; 149: 33–37.
Normal	Re-establishes BF as the norm; de-normalizes artificial feeding.	Koop, C. Everett, MD. *Report of the Surgeon General's Workshop on Breastfeeding and Human Lactation.* Washington, D.C.: National Center for Education in Maternal and Child Health, 1984. Baumslag N, Michels DL. *Milk, Money and Madness: the Culture and Politics of Breastfeeding.* Westport, CT: Bergin and Garvey, 1995.
Reassuring	Bonding and closeness are unique advantages of BF. BF fosters the emotional development of mothers and babies.	Thoman, Evelyn B., Browder Sue. *Born Dancing: How Intuitive Parents Understand Their Baby's Unspoken Language and Natural Rhythms.* New York: Harper and Row, 1987. Klaus, Marshall H., Kennell, John H. *Parent-infant Bonding, Second Edition.* St. Louis: C.V. Mosby, 1982.

Breastfeeding (BF) Is...	Teaching Points	References
Relaxing	Mother and baby are stressed when separated. Lactation enhances Mom's ability to cope with stress. Baby and Mom relax during feedings.	Altemus M, Deuster PA, et al. Suppression of hypothalamus-pituitary-adrenal axis responses to stress in lactating women. *Journal of Clinical Endocrinology and Metabolism* 1995; 80: 2954–59. Uvnas-Moberg, Kerstin. The gastrointestinal tract in growth and reproduction. *Scientific American*, July 1989: 78–83.
Safe	Mother's own milk is the safest food for baby. Breasts are the safest devices for feeding, and Mom protects baby when BF.	Lawrence, Ruth A. *Breastfeeding, a Guide for the Medical Profession, Fifth Edition.* St. Louis: Mosby, 1999. Minchin, Maureen. *Breastfeeding Matters: What We Need to Know about Infant Feeding, Fourth Revised Edition.* St. Kilda, Australia: Alma Publications, 1998.
Satisfying	BF is pleasurable and gratifying for mother as she fulfills part of her rich biological role.	Newton, Niles. *Maternal Emotions.* New York: Harper & Brothers, 1955. Kitzinger, Sheila. *Woman as Mothers: How They See Themselves in Different Cultures.* New York: Random House, 1978.

continues

continued

Breastfeeding (BF) Is. . .	Teaching Points	References
Smart	Breastfeeding fosters brain development, improves I.Q., vision, and nerve function. Milk components and the mothering during BF are both critical factors.	Lucas A, Morley R, Cole TJ, Lister G, Lesson-Payne C. Breastmilk and subsequent intelligence quotient in children born preterm. *Lancet* 1992; 339: 261–64. Uauy R, DeAndraca I. Human milk and breastfeeding for optimal mental development. *Journal of Nutrition* 1995; Vol 125 supplement: 2,278–2,280.
Timeless	Babies were biologically programmed to breast-feed for two to seven years. Historical evidence is strong for extended BF.	Fildes, Valerie. *Breasts, Bottles and Babies: a History of Infant Feeding.* Edinburgh: Edinburgh University Press, 1986. Stuart-Macadam P, Dettwyler KA (eds). *Breastfeeding: Biocultural Perspectives.* New York: Aldine De Gruyter, 1995.
Wonderful	Some mothers BF *against all odds* partly because BF is so phe-nomenal.	Botroff, J. L. Persistence in breastfeeding: a phenomenological investigation. *Journal of Advanced Nursing* 15 (1990): 201–209. Best Start, Inc. *Breastfeeding: For all the Right Reasons.* Tampa: Best Start, Inc., 1990.

BREASTFEEDING QUIZ

· ·

GOAL

To present research-based facts about benefits of breastfeeding and risks of artificial feeding in an interesting format.

BEST AUDIENCE

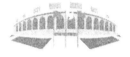

Any

TIME REQUIRED

10–20 minutes

HOW TO PLAY

This game can be played by creating a handout with the following questions or by asking the questions one at a time to an audience. Be prepared to discuss the answers, and to provide references as needed.

Question	Answer

1. In the United States, how many deaths from diarrhea are attributed yearly to artificial feeding?
 	
   a. 50–100
   b. 100–250
   c. 250–300
   d. 400–500
	c. **250–300.** In developing countries and in situations/locations with poor sanitary conditions, the death rates associated with artificial feeding are even higher.

continues

continued

Question	Answer
2. Which of the following gastrointestinal diseases are NOT associated with artificial feeding? **a.** Crohn's disease **b.** Inflammatory bowel disease **c.** Celiac disease **d.** Duodenal ulcers	**d. Duodenal ulcers.** Occurrences of all of the other diseases are higher in people who were not breastfed.
3. Which of the following statements regarding otitis media is FALSE? **a.** Artificially-fed babies have double the rate of ear infections than babies who are breastfed. **b.** Artificially-fed babies have more recurrent ear infections than babies who are breastfed. **c.** The feeding method does not affect the rate of ear infections. **d.** The cost to treat ear infections is higher for artificially-fed children.	**c. The feeding method does not affect the rate of ear infections is FALSE.** In one analysis, otitis media increases medical costs by an average of $30 per child per year.
4. Compared to breastfed babies, artificially-fed babies have how much increased risk of contracting bacteremia and meningitis? **a.** Two times **b.** Three times **c.** Four times **d.** Five times	**c. Four times.** These diseases are serious illnesses, which often result in hospitalization.

Question	Answer

5. *Not* breastfeeding and exposure to formula are attributed to how much of an increased risk of acquiring juvenile insulin-dependent diabetes?
 	
  a. 10 percent
  b. 15 percent
  c. 20 percent
  d. 25 percent
	d. **25 percent.** Non-insulin–dependent diabetes is also associated with *not* having been breastfed.

6. Artificially-fed children have how much increased risk of childhood (up to 15 years) malignant lymphomas?
 	
  a. Two to four times
  b. Four to six times
  c. Six to eight times
  d. Eight to ten times
	c. **Six to eight times.** This increased risk also applies to Hodgkin's disease.

7. Women over 40 who were breastfed as children have how much LESS a risk for breast cancer?
 	
  a. 10 percent
  b. 15 percent
  c. 20 percent
  d. 25 percent
	d. **25 percent less.** Breastfeeding also reduces breast cancer risk for those women who breastfeed their children.

8. Protection against multiple sclerosis in adults is associated with
 	
  a. Being breastfed one month
  b. Being breastfed six months
  c. Being breastfed four months
  d. Ever being breastfed
	c. **Being breastfed four months longer than controls.** The fatty acids in human milk appear to have a protective effect against several neurological conditions.

continues

continued

Question	Answer
9. Which statement about allergic disease being related to feeding method is FALSE? a. 42 percent of gastroesophageal reflux is related to cow milk allergy. b. Breastfed children have a delayed onset of allergic disease. c. Breastfeeding prevents allergies. d. Breastfed children have less wheezing.	c. **Breastfeeding prevents allergies.** Allergic disease is inherited. Breastfeeding delays the onset and lessens the severity of allergic responses in children, especially in families in which one or both parents are allergic.
10. All of the following diseases are positively associated with artificial feeding EXCEPT a. Muscular dystrophy b. Chronic respiratory disease c. Coronary artery disease d. Higher cholesterol in young adulthood	a. **Muscular dystrophy.** As of December 2000, no research has addressed the possible links between muscular dystrophy and infant feeding methods.
11. Which nutrient is LEAST LIKELY to improve cognitive and neurological development? a. Lactose b. Long-chain polyunsaturated fatty acids c. Proteins d. Lactoferrin	d. **Lactoferrin.** Lactose is strongly associated with cognitive function; long-chain polyunsaturated fatty acids are associated with I.Q. improvement; and human milk protein is predominately whey, which fosters alertness.

Question	Answer
12. Higher cognitive and neuromotor test scores of children in middle-income families are LEAST LIKELY to be related to a. Length of exclusive breastfeeding b. Age when solids were introduced c. Ever having been breastfed d. Duration of breastfeeding	**b. Age when solids were introduced.** These differences are still measurable in middle school children by teachers and parents and have been documented since the 1920s.
13. When tested at ages seven to eight years, premature babies who received their mother's milk through a feeding tube had which of the following, compared to artificially-fed premature babies? a. Five points higher I.Q. b. 10 points higher I.Q. c. Same I.Q. d. 15 points higher I.Q.	**b. 10 points higher I.Q.** Dr. Alan Lucas controlled the many variables in this landmark research.
14. Human milk improves all of the following neuromotor functions EXCEPT a. Hearing b. Deficits realted to congenital cretinism c. Visual acuity d. Neuromotor skills in impaired children	**a. Hearing.** No research to date has looked at the possible links between hearing and feeding methods. The other improvements are positively associated with breastfeeding.

continues

continued

Question	Answer

15. Human milk and breastfeeding has which of the following effects on dental health?
 	
  a. More decay in primary teeth
  b. No effects
  c. Less orthodontia
  d. Weaker muscles of mastication (chewing)
	c. Less orthodontia. Artificial feeding is associated with weaker muscles of mastication and more need for orthodontia. No solid association has been found between extended nighttime feeding and baby-bottle tooth decay.

16. Which of the following would a breastfeeding woman expect in the postpartum period?
 	
  a. Increased postpartum bleeding
  b. Slow uterine involution
  c. Difficulty returning to pre-pregnant weight
  d. Delayed return of menstruation and fertility
	d. Delayed return of menstruation and fertility. Globally, the Lactational Amennorrhea Method (LAM) of family planning prevents more unplanned pregnancies than all of the other methods combined.

17. Maternal benefits of breastfeeding extend past the childbearing age. Which of the following are NOT related to breastfeeding?
 	
  a. Reduced risk of hip fractures
  b. Reduced risk of ovarian cancer
  c. Reduced risk of premenopausal breast cancer
  d. Earlier menopause
	d. Earlier menopause. All the other reductions are strongly correlated to lactation.

Question	Answer

18. Economic benefits of breastfeeding include all of the following EXCEPT
 	
  a. Increased costs for special breastfeeding garments
  b. Reduced health care costs
  c. Reduced employee absenteeism to care for sick infants
  d. Reduced expenses for infant formula in the WIC program
	a. Increased cost for special breastfeeding garments. Mothers can wear ordinary clothing while breastfeeding, although some purchase special garments. The other economic benefits are documented.

19. What is the risk of fatal or nonfatal respiratory infection in artificially-fed babies?
 	
  a. None
  b. Two to five times
  c. Three to eight times
  d. Greater than 10 times
	b. Two to five times. The increased risk for respiratory infections includes bronchitis, pneumonia, upper and lower airway infections, and wheezing, along with their related expenses.

20. Who was the first U.S. president to be born in a hospital?
 	
  a. Harry Truman
  b. Jimmy Carter
  c. Bill Clinton
  d. William Harding
	b. Jimmy Carter. All the U.S. presidents prior to Jimmy Carter were born at home.

Adapted from the following sources:

* *The Curriculum in Support of the Ten Steps to Successful Breastfeeding: An 18 Hour Interdisciplinary Breastfeeding Management Course for the United States,* U.S. Department of Health and Human Services, Maternal and Child Health Bureau, January 1999.

* *Fact Packs 1–6,* Bright Future Lactation Resource Center 1993–1998, www.bflrc.com.

4

DRILLS AND LEAD-UP GAMES

Activities for
Learning Specific
Principles and Skills

BREASTMILK BIOCHEMISTRY BINGO[1]

GOAL

To teach information on milk composition, biochemistry, and immunology in an interactive manner

BEST AUDIENCE

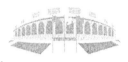

Health care professionals and lactation management students. For this game, the instructor must have a deep and thorough knowledge of the subject matter in order to answer technical or scientific questions that may be posed by students.

TIME REQUIRED

90 minutes

HOW TO PLAY

1. Purchase or make a set of Bingo cards and markers. Most commercially available cards have 75 numbers, so use only 75 statement cards. Bingo cards with more numbers can also be created using computer programs. If you make your own cards, laminate them for longer wear.

2. Make up *statement cards* that contain one fact per card. One way to create them is to print the facts on printer-ready labels and then stick the labels onto index cards.

3. Distribute one bingo card and a set of markers to each student. Small peel-off stickers can be used as markers on laminated cards. Have students remove the stickers from their cards after the game so you do not get stuck removing all of them yourself. A teachers' store or office supply store should have a selection of inexpensive stickers available.

---

[1] **Source:** This game was originally developed for the *Lactation Consultant Exam Preparation Course* formerly taught through Lact-Ed, Inc.

4. Set out the bingo goals and prizes. The *first* person to get each bingo wins a prize. Eventually everyone should have a full card. Make sure that everyone eventually gets at least one prize. (Prizes could be breastfeeding postcards, note cards, bumper stickers, specially-imprinted pens, pin-on breastfeeding theme buttons, candy treats, and so forth.) Players can win with any of the following bingos:

    a. First bingo in any direction

    b. First vertical bingo

    c. First horizontal bingo

    d. First diagonal bingo

    e. All four corners

    f. Full card covered

5. Shuffle and read one statement card at a time, allowing students enough time to find and cover the corresponding number on their bingo cards. Or, deal or pass out the statement cards and have students take turns reading one statement at a time. Although having students read the cards takes longer, it keeps them more interested in the facts. Expand upon any of the statements that seem confusing or have *and furthermore* implications.

6. Remind students not to try and memorize the statements as they are read, but to simply play the game and get a sense of the extraordinary uniqueness of human milk. Provide them with a printed list of the statements for further reference and refer them to texts with more information. If any of the biological or chemical terms are unfamiliar to students, the instructor should briefly explain the term and remind the students to read (or re-read) more about human milk biochemistry in lactation textbooks.

    Teaching tip: Assemble some plastic interlocking pop beads into an interesting shape to illustrate a molecule of one of the protective proteins, say lactoferrin. In its original shape, the molecule functions as lactoferrin. Digestion, freezing, or disturbing the molecule may break it into peptide fragments (you break apart the beads), which are then digested as nutrients. You get two results for the price of one. With infant formula, all the baby gets is the fragments.

    Teaching tip: You might also bring some Lego® building blocks and partly assemble them into a shape. Leave some blocks on the table. Tell the group "This game is going to examine individual blocks (or information about milk components) in detail. We are not going to assemble them today, so do not agonize over the implications of this information just yet—simply allow yourself to examine the details of each block."

SAMPLE BREASTMILK BIOCHEMISTRY STATEMENTS

Note: Use any or all of the following list as needed.

1. Mature human milk consists of about 0.9 percent protein.

2. Humans are a frequent-contact species.

3. Each mammal's milk components are specific to that species.

4. Human milk is 99 percent bioavailable.

5. The whey:casein ratio of human milk averages 80:20; it varies from 90:10 early in lactation to 60:40 as the baby gets older.

6. Cow's milk protein is 82 percent casein and 18 percent whey.

7. Human casein forms soft, small, easily digestible curds.

8. Colostrum is very dense—almost gel-like.

9. Colostrum is a low-volume feed.

10. Colostrum is lower in lactose than mature milk.

11. Colostrum facilitates the passage of meconium and is rich in antioxidants.

12. Colostrum is lower in water-soluble vitamins than mature milk.

13. Colostrum is higher in protein than the same volume of mature milk.

14. Colostrum is higher in fat-soluble vitamins than mature milk.

15. Colostrum is higher in sodium, potassium, and chloride than mature milk.

16. Colostrum is higher in zinc than mature milk.

17. Colostrum's yellow color comes from beta-carotene and other caretenoids.

18. Colostrum is high in immunoglobulins.

19. High-volume feeds in the first few days of life stress the newborn's immature kidneys.

20. Immunoglobulins coat the gut lining to prevent adherence of pathogens.

21. The protein content of human milk is the lowest of all mammalian milks. High-protein feeds are associated with increased illness.

22. Many milk constituents serve dual roles. For example, alpha-lactalbumin supplies amino acids to the infant and helps transport calcium and zinc.

continues

continued

23. Human milk has a low solute load, which is easier on immature kidneys.

24. Human whey is predominantly of alpha-lactalbumin.

25. The beta-lactoglobulin of cow's milk is responsible for antigenic (allergic) responses in humans.

26. Human milk contains taurine, which is important for fat absorption and central nervous system (CNS) development, and is now considered an essential amino acid for children.

27. Lactoferrin is produced in the milk ducts and may be one of the factors that protects breastfeeding mothers from later ductal cancers.

28. Lactoferrin is the iron-binding protein found in whey. Because human milk is about 80 percent whey, lactoferrin is found in abundance.

29. Lactoferrin robs gut pathogens of the iron they need to proliferate.

30. Fatty acids (including DHA and AA), lactose, hormones, and growth factors in human milk affect psychomotor development.

31. Colostrum has 2g (.07 ounces)/100ml (3.38 ounces) of fat, mature milk has 4 (.01 ounces)–4.5g (.16 ounces)/100ml (3.38 ounces) of fat.

32. Fatty acids in milk derive partly from maternal diet and mostly from the mother's fat stores.

33. Fat levels in human milk vary during the 24-hour day and are related to the relative fullness or emptiness of the breast.

34. Ninety-eight percent of all lipids in human milk are enclosed in globules.

35. Triglycerides dominate lipid composition.

36. The membranes of fat globules are made up of phospholipids, sterols (especially cholesterol), and proteins.

37. The fatty-acid composition of breastmilk is relatively stable—42 percent saturated and 57 percent unsaturated.

38. Maternal diet can influence the proportions of certain types of polyunsaturated fatty acids including linoleic, linolenic, and other long chain fatty acids.

39. Fatty acids are essential for proper CNS development, including brain growth and nerve myelination.

40. Cholesterol levels are stable in human milk and cannot be manipulated by maternal diet changes.

41. Both unsaturated and saturated fatty acids are important to brain development.

42. Lactose is essential for lactogenesis and ongoing milk synthesis, and directly influences milk volume.

43. Lactose is the dominant sugar found in human milk. Other sugars are galactose, fructose, and oligosaccharides.

44. Colostrum has 4 percent lactose. Mature milk has 7 percent lactose.

45. Lactase, the enzyme that metabolizes lactose, is found only in infant mammals. Lactase is present in humans for at least two to seven years.

46. Lactose assists in the absorption of calcium and iron.

47. Lactose is a constituent of the galactolipids, which are needed for CNS development.

48. Lactose and other sugars supply at least 40 percent of the infant's energy needs.

49. Lactose promotes infant intestinal colonization with Lactobacillus bifidus.

50. The concentrations of iron, copper, and zinc are especially high in colostrum and gradually decline. Levels of these minerals in human milk are not related to maternal diet.

51. Water-soluble vitamin levels in human milk can vary with maternal intake.

52. The fat-soluble vitamin content follows the variations of fat levels in milk and is somewhat affected by maternal diet.

53. The concentration of vitamin K is higher in colostrum and early milk until vitamin K is manufactured in the infant gut in the first weeks postpartum.

54. The concentration of vitamin A is two times higher in colostrum than in mature milk and is higher in human milk than in cow milk.

55. Vitamin E is found in adequate amounts in human milk.

56. Human milk contains low concentrations of vitamin D which is found in both fat and aqueous fractions of milk.

57. Ideally, vitamin D is obtained via skin absorption. A week's worth of vitamin D can be absorbed from 10 minutes of full body exposure or from 30 minutes of head and hand exposure in the sunlight.

58. Long-chain polyunsaturated fatty acids (DHA and AA) in human milk are critical for brain and cognitive development, vision, and nerve myelinization.

59. Mothers who are well nourished have adequate amounts of water-soluble vitamins in their milk. Case reports of vitamin deficiencies in breastfed infants are rare.

60. Most minerals remain stable in human milk regardless of maternal diet.

continues

continued

61. Up to 70 percent of iron in human milk is utilized by the infant, due to complex mechanisms governing iron absorption.

62. Lactoferrin acts as an iron transfer agent.

63. Healthy term infants have enough hepatic (liver) stores of iron to meet their needs for up to 12 months.

64. Iron supplementation (through vitamin drops or early solids) carries substantial risks to the infant by binding lactoferrin and feeding pathogens.

65. The exclusively breastfed infant is at little risk of having either a deficiency or excess of trace elements, including fluorine.

66. Copper, selenium, chromium, manganese, molybdenum, and nickel are trace elements in milk that are critical to growth and development. Some of these elements are considered essential nutrients.

67. Human milk contains hormonally active peptides including epidermal growth factor (EGF) and nerve growth factor (NGF). Researchers are just beginning to understand the role that growth factors have in infant development.

68. Immunofactors IgA, IgM, IgG; lysozyme and other enzymes; lactoferrin; and bifidus factor are soluble components in the whey fraction of human milk.

69. Macrophages, lymphocytes, neutrophils, and epithelial cells are cellular components of human milk.

70. Immunofactors are high in colostrum, decrease in mature milk, and rise high again in regression milk so that intakes remain constant throughout lactation.

71. Secretory IgA (SigA) is the most important immunofactor of human milk. SIgA coats the gut and binds pathogens to it.

72. An exclusively breastfed infant receives at least 0.5 gm (.02 ounces) of SIgA per day in the first month of life, which is 50 times the dose given to a patient with hypoglobulinemia.

73. SIgA is secreted in the intestinal tract and is produced in the mammary gland. It is present in high concentration in the first week of life after birth, falling to a stable level of about 2 mg/ml in mature milk.

74. Starting supplements or solids (and even pacifiers) introduces pathogens and allergens to the baby and also binds lactoferrin.

75. Human milk stimulates the infant's own production of SIgA.

76. Lactoferrin is bacteriostatic because it binds to iron, thus starving the pathogenic bacteria in the gut.

77. Lactoferrin promotes intestinal colonization with lactobaccilli in the presence of lactose.

78. Lactoferrin prevents the growth of E. coli and fungi.

79. Lactoferrin plays an active role in the prevention of necrotizing enterocolitis (NEC). NEC is gangrene of the gut tissues.

80. Cellular immunofactors are phagocytic and secrete immune substances that are specific to microorganisms with which the mother has come into contact.

81. Human milk contains viral fragments which cannot be replicated and which stimulate antibody responses in infants.

82. Mucins in human milk bind with and destroy pathogens.

83. Bifidus factor is a carbohydrate that helps maintain colonization of the gut with Lactobacillus bifidus, a beneficial organism.

84. Human milk composition varies from day to day, from mother to mother, between breasts, between feeds, in a single feed, in the short term, and over the long term.

85. Milk from mothers who give birth prematurely is uniquely suited for their preterm babies.

86. Preterm milk contains higher levels of immunoglobulins, lysozyme, lactoferrin, and white cells than mature milk.

87. Mother's own milk matches 50 percent of the baby's genetic material.

88. Pooled, pasteurized donor human milk for a premature baby may need added zinc because zinc levels decrease over the duration of lactation. A mother's own milk has sufficient zinc for her infant.

89. Maternal fluid intake is unrelated to the volume of milk produced. Overhydration of 25 percent may reduce milk volume.

90. Anti-inflammatory agents in human milk double as direct protective agents, anti-oxidants, and enzymes.

91. Green milk can be caused by the intake of chlorophyll or by mammary duct ectasia. It is considered safe for the baby.

92. Proteins, carbohydrates, and lipids in milk are synthesized in the mammary gland and transferred from maternal plasma to milk.

93. Pink milk is usually milk that has blood in it. It is considered safe for the baby, although the source of the blood should be investigated.

continues

continued

94. Mean secretion volume of colostrum is 30 ml (1.01 ounces)/day. The range is 10 (.338 ounces) to 100 ml (3.38 ounces)/day.

95. Increased fluid volume and carbohydrate levels in milk begin 30–40 hours post-birth, initiating the changes in milk composition from colostrum to mature milk.

96. Regression milk resembles colostrum in its high levels of immunoglobulins, which protect both the weaning baby and the breast itself.

97. Epidermal growth factor is a potent peptide in human milk, which helps mature the infant lungs and gastrointestinal tract and promotes DNA synthesis.

98. The dominant protein in bovine milk is beta-lactoglobulin, which has no human milk counterpart.

99. Prostaglandins in human milk aid intestinal motility, have a protective effect on the bowel, and are important to digestion and gut maturation.

100. Hormones present in human milk include oxytocin, prolactin, adrenal and ovarian steroids, relaxin, and insulin.

Eating Patterns (Golf Ball) Game

GOAL

To fully appreciate infant nutritional needs and the need for frequent feedings

BEST AUDIENCE
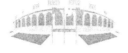

Groups of at least 10 people—parents or professionals

TIME REQUIRED

10–20 minutes

HOW TO PLAY

There are two parts to this game.

Part One:

Everyone needs pencil and paper, which will not be collected. Instructor says to the students:

"Think about a day that you had reasonably free access to food (for example, use today if the class is during the evening). Write down the time whenever you ate or drank anything—even water counts. Count drinking from fountains, brushing your teeth, coffee breaks, snacks, and meals. Put a star by the meals, write down the length of time the meals took, and the average time between eating or drinking episodes. Next, draw a diagram of the size of a newborn infant's stomach (it should be 50 cc, or golf-ball size). Then somewhere on your paper, figure out what your weight would be, if doubled, and name a prize you would dearly love to win—the more extravagant the better. Finally, write down several words that describe how you feel when you are truly hungry or thirsty and do not have access to food or drink."

Then ask the students the following questions:

1. How often did you eat? (Answers will average every one to three hours).

2. How long did the meals take? (Answers will average 20–30 minutes).

3. Why would you ever want to take longer than this to eat a meal? (Answers will include conversation, social time, relaxing, and so forth.)

4. How do you feel if you are truly hungry or thirsty and cannot get food or water? Does skipping a meal teach you to go longer without food or make you more desperate for food?

5. Are you trying to gain weight? (This question results in laughter, of course.)

6. To earn your prize, all you have to do is double your weight in five months. What will you do differently from what you are now doing?

The answers offered will be easy to correlate to infant needs—eat more often/constantly/ at night; eat higher calorie food (hindmilk); do not postpone meals; do not drink water in place of eating; take time at meals; avoid exercise, and so on.

Then display or toss someone a golf ball to illustrate the size of a baby's stomach. Remind students that there are no calories in a pacifier.

Comment that there is never an advantage to keeping a baby hungry when he or she needs to eat, and only the baby can determine her own hunger and appetite.

This part of the discussion can be expanded by asking, "What utensil did you use to eat?" "What if you had to use your nondominant hand and a different utensil, such as chopsticks?" These questions will lead students into a discussion of the consequences of feeding difficulties associated with using artificial teats and other sucking objects.

Note: This game always works. I have had tremendous success with it in every kind of group, from teenagers to physicians. I love the responses to "How do you feel when you're hungry?"

Part Two:

To set up the game, ask for three volunteers from the audience. One volunteer will be the *victim* in the accident; one will be the *nice caretaker*; and one will be the *clueless caretaker*. Coach each player in their respective roles (see following text). Next, place a chair in the front, facing the audience. Have the victim sit in the chair, introduce the following story, and have the voluteers begin acting.

The victim was skiing in the mountains of Peru (any country where English is not the primary language will work in this game). She caught her ski in a tree root, tumbled down a cliff, and landed in a twisted heap. After being rescued, she is now in the local hospital with two broken legs and two broken arms, and her face is swollen so much that she cannot even open her mouth. It is now several hours later, and she is getting hungry and thirsty but cannot speak the local language, and even if she could, her face is swollen shut.

The first (clueless) caretaker comes in to take care of the victim. Instruct the victim by stating, "Try to tell the caretaker that you are hungry and thirsty. Remember, you have two broken legs and two broken arms, and your face is swollen shut." The clueless caretaker has been coached to *ignore and misinterpret the victim's signals and to be as perfunctory as possible in tending to the victim.* Allow this situation to play itself out for a few minutes until it is clear that the victim is becoming more and more desperate to get food and water, and the caretaker is simply not responsive to the victim's needs.

The clueless caretaker now leaves, and the nice caretaker comes in. Repeat your previous instructions. This time, however, the nice caretaker *immediately understands the victim's gestures and sounds, figures out how to provide water and edible food to the victim, fluffs her pillow, wipes her face with a cool cloth, anticipates other needs, and so on.* Allow this situation to play itself out for a few minutes until the victim's relief is clear.

Finally, to wrap up the game, thank the volunteers for their participation. Ask each, "What was it like to play that role?" Then ask the victim what would happen if the tables were turned—if the victim were to become the caretaker for the two others, who are injured or ill and under her care.

Correlate this discussion to infant cues for feeding; the long-term trust that is built when mother anticipates and responds to a baby's feeding cues; and the negative consequences when feeding cues are repeatedly ignored and misinterpreted.

Variations of the game:

* I would suggest for a class/group to feed the mamas. There's something about a snack that makes coming and chatting a bit more interesting. I think adults like to talk over food.

  —Pierrette Mimi Poinsett, MD, FAAP; Modesto, CA

* After they have a snack, that's a perfect opportunity to point out that they took the food even though they're not trying to gain weight, that they didn't need it but derived pleasure from it anyway, that they felt more comfortable and cared for because of it—in short, that they needn't try to gauge whether their little one "is hungry yet" before offering the breast as a solution to whatever is making him wiggly.

  —Diane Wiessinger, MS, IBCLC; Ithaca, NY

* Pass around a bowl of *wrapped* chocolates or candy (I did this with chocolate kisses.) Before the participants have had a chance to unwrap them, cry "STOP! You can only have a candy if you have not eaten anything else within the last two hours!" Now watch their faces. Another version of this is to pass around the candy once without comment, and a few minutes later pass it again. Ask why they took the first piece (so soon after lunch, etc.) Ask who took a second piece . . . or a third . . . or one for later . . .

  —Norma Ritter, IBCLC; Big Flats, NY

FIGURES DON'T LIE: EVALUATING BREASTFEEDING RESEARCH[2]

GOAL

To identify the pertinent elements in research designs and to learn how to dissect and evaluate published research pertinent to breastfeeding

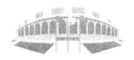

BEST AUDIENCE

Health care professionals and lactation management students. For this game, the instructor must have a deep and thorough knowledge of the subject matter in order to answer technical or scientific questions that may be posed by students.

TIME REQUIRED

90 minutes

HOW TO PLAY

Prepare by collecting several research articles that are relevant to breastfeeding and lactation. Each student should have their own article to read; however, several students may have the same article. Follow international copyright law in obtaining these articles.

Part One:

Allow about 20 minutes for students to read their articles and to identify the following components:

1. Problem statement and/or hypothesis

2. Literature review

3. Target population or sample

---

[2]**Source:** This game was originally developed for the *Lactation Consultant Exam Preparation Course* formerly taught through Lact-Ed, Inc.

4. Study design

5. Data collection, analysis, and statistical tests

6. Findings/results

7. Discussion and conclusion

8. Graphics—graphs, charts, or photographs

Part Two:

Have students read the articles again (allow about 20–30 minutes). Students with the same article can work together. Have students look for the following common flaws:

* Poor, inadequate operational definitions—especially for "breastfed," "normal suck," "normal birth," and so forth.

* Inappropriate study design

* The mixing of artificial feeding and breastfeeding in the subjects and controls

* Funding sources with conflict of interest

* The drawing of conclusions not based on evidence

Have students analyze the article thoroughly and report the following information back to the large group:

1. What was studied and/or reported on

2. Any flaws found

3. Whether the student would advise changing clinical practice on the basis of the article's findings

4. Any other additional comments

End the session by summarizing and recapping the key research concepts.

Some suggested research articles for this game follow. Other research articles can also be used. Include at least one randomized controlled trial, one qualitative design, a flawed article, and one with a sound design and important conclusions:

Aarts C, Hornell A, Kylberg E, Hofvander Y, Gebre-Medhin M. Breastfeeding patterns in relation to thumb sucking and pacifier use. *Pediatrics* 1999; 104(4): e50. or www.pediatrics.org/cgi/content/full/104/4/e50.

Ball TM, Wright AL. Health care costs of formula-feeding in the first year of life. *Pediatrics* 1999; 103: 870–876.

Cronenwett L, Stukel T, Kearney M, Barrett J, Covington C, Del Monte K, Reinhardt R, Rippe L. Single daily bottle use in the early weeks postpartum and breastfeeding outcomes. *Pediatrics* 1992; 90(5): 760–766.

Crowell MK, Hill PD, Humenick, SS. Relationship between obstetric analgesia and time of effective breastfeeding. *J Nurse-Midwifery* May/June 1994; 39(3): 150–156.

Gray L, Watt L, Blass EM. Skin-to-skin contact is analgesic in healthy newborns. *Pediatrics* 2000; 105(1): e14, or www.Pediatrics.org/cgi/content/full/105/1/e14.

Halpern SH, Levine T, Wilson DB, et al. Effect of labor analgesia on breastfeeding success. *Birth* 1999; 26(2): 83–88.

Kennell J, Klaus M, McGrath S, Robertson S, Hinkley C. Continuous emotional support during labor in a U.S. hospital. A randomized controlled trial. *JAMA* 1991; 265(17): 2197–2201.

Locklin MP, Naber, SJ. Does breastfeeding empower women? Insights from a select group of educated, low-income, minority women. *Birth* 1993; 20(1): 30–35.

Loftus J, Hill H, Cohen S: Placental transfer and neonatal effects of epidural sufentanil and fentanyl administered with bupivicaine during labor. *Anesthesiology* 1995; 83: 300–308.

Meier P, Anderson GC. Responses of small preterm infants to bottle- and breastfeeding. *MCN* March/April 1987; 12: 97–103.

Righard L, Alade, MO. Effect of delivery room routines on success of first breastfeed. *Lancet* 1990; 336: 1105–1107.

Sepkoski CM, Lester BM, Ostheimer GW, Brazelton TB. The effect of maternal epidural anesthesia on neonatal behavior during the first month. *Developmental Medicine and Child Neurology* 1992; 34: 1072–1080.

How To Talk so Mothers Will Listen and Listen so Mothers Will Talk, or Listening Between the Lines[3]

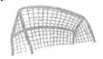

GOAL

To help breastfeeding care providers acquire effective counseling skills for breastfeeding situations—that is, how to "listen so mothers will talk and talk so mothers will listen."

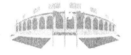

BEST AUDIENCE

Health care professionals and lactation management students. There should be at least one instructor who is experienced in this counseling technique/style for every eight to twelve students.

TIME REQUIRED

90–120 minutes with 10–15 minutes for a break midway through the game

HOW TO PLAY

To prepare for the game, create a set of about 100 *statement cards*—using the list provided later in the text. (One way to create the cards is to print the statements on printer-ready labels, and then stick the labels onto index cards.) Provide each student a copy of a *feeling word* vocabulary, which is provided later in the text. Include statements that reflect a wide variety of situations and emotions from mothers, family members, professional colleagues, physicians, and coworkers.

To begin, divide the group so that eight to twelve students work with one instructor. If possible, each group should be isolated from the others to reduce noise and to improve the emotional aspect of the game. If only one instructor is available, then divide the group into teams of eight to twelve and circulate from group to group

---

[3] **Source:** This game was adapted from La Leche League International's *Human Relations Enrichment, Level 1* program for use in the *Lactation Consultant Exam Preparation Course* formerly taught through Lact-Ed, Inc.

during the exercise. Teams should sit in a circle or around a table. Distribute the statement cards so that each student has several.

Part 1: Equivalent responses

Introduce the concept of *addressing the speaker's feelings* before beginning to solve the problem. Introduce the *you feel . . . because* pattern. Explain how to use this word structure model and the *feeling word* list.

Next, ask someone to read (or make up) a statement and demonstrate the patterned response at an equivalent level of emotion. For example, "My mother keeps on nagging me to use a pacifier. She just won't let go of that idea no matter what I say to her." You respond by saying, "You feel frustrated that your mother continues to suggest pacifiers, even when you've told her your views." Repeat this pattern three to five times, using several different statements.

Then have the teams practice this step. Distribute the statement cards and have each group sit in a circle. One person will read or invent a statement, and the person seated next to her responds. The responder will then read or invent a statement, and the next person in the circle will respond. If the responder has trouble formulating a response, wait a bit before inviting the group members to suggest a response.

For each statement, continue until the speaker feels that her emotions have been acknowledged and she is ready to begin solving the problem or discussing the facts of the situation. The responses can move into a more conversational format as long as the feeling (emotion) of the speaker is named by the responder.

Continue this pattern for about 20–30 minutes or until every student has read or invented at least three statements and has had an opportunity to respond to at least three statements.

Note: The instructor may need to clarify or remind students that this exercise is *not about solving the clinical problem*—it is about *validating the speaker's feelings* before moving on to solving the problem. Some statements may require several exchanges before the speaker feels she has been *heard* enough to move on to problem solving. Sometimes exploring the speaker's feelings is sufficient to resolve this situation. Encourage as many exchanges—statements and responses—as necessary until the speaker feels she has been heard. After a few rounds of the *you feel . . . because* template, a more conversational sentence structure can be used as long as the responder uses a feeling word or clearly identifies the emotion(s) behind the statement being spoken.

Part 2: Additive responses

Next, introduce the concept of additive responses which focus even more on the feeling and explore the reason for that feeling in more detail or depth. Ask students to read a few statements and demonstrate the patterned response with an additive level of response. For example, "My mother keeps on nagging me to use a pacifier. She just won't let go of that idea no matter what I say to her." Additive response: "You are furious because she insists that her idea is the right one. Her behavior must be particularly maddening because you researched the pros and cons of pacifiers before making made your decision. You feel angry, disappointed, and hurt because your mother seems determined to second guess your mothering decision."

Then collect and redistribute the statement cards so that each person gets some new statements to use. Once again, statements can be invented. Repeat the first exercise using additive responses for each statement this time.

Some statement and response exchanges may have to go back and forth several times before the original speaker feels they have been fully heard and is ready to move on. This round may take longer than the previous one because the *background* for each response must be invented on the spot.

Continue this pattern for about 20–30 minutes or until every student has read or invented at least three statements and has had an opportunity to respond to at least three statements.

Conclusion:

Reassemble the large group and summarize the philosophy behind this style of counseling. Ask them what they learned, and how it can be applied.

Resources:

The vocabulary list on page 86 includes many, but not all, words used to describe feelings. The descriptions of intensity levels may differ from your own. Feel free to add other words to the list.

The following statements are samples that can be used in this game:

STATEMENTS

....

* I just can't get anything done. All I do is carry that baby around all day. He's fussy all the time.

* I just couldn't wait to come and tell you! I'm finally pregnant!

* That night nurse really messed us up by giving Sara a bottle of formula. Now she keeps wanting to nurse on the tip of my nipple.

* My doctor said he believes most mothers can give birth vaginally after they've had a cesarean. . . I found out later that he has never done a VBAC!

* I thought breastfeeding would really tie me down. Now I love it as much as the baby does!

---

continues

continued

* My sister went on and on about my being a Jersey cow because I nurse Holly so often.

* I picked my doctor because she is supposedly supportive of breastfeeding, yet she insists that I give my baby water after I nurse.

* My husband is a pain right now. He gets mad if the house is a mess when he gets home, yet does nothing to help when he's around.

* Those teenagers who keep having babies really aggravate me. They should have their tubes tied if they can't support their kids!

* These new consent forms are stupid! I spend more time filling them out than taking care of the babies in the nursery.

* The new formula representative really does support breastfeeding. Look at all these videos he gave us!

* That speaker's opinion that pacifiers are harmful is just plain nonsense. I used one, and my baby is just fine.

* I need to rent a pump because my doctor wants to see how much milk I'm making. He said that Nathan isn't gaining enough weight.

* I've read that breastfeeding is really better for the baby, but I couldn't possibly do it in public.

* Why did that doctor tell me I had to stop nursing during a breast infection? My baby and I were both miserable, and now she won't take my breast.

* That new head nurse burns me up with her insistence on no water bottles in the cribs.

* That mother in Room 5B says she will start breastfeeding when she gets home because the first milk is bad for the baby.

* That last patient claims she wants to breastfeed, yet she gives me an argument for everything I suggest.

* I don't think I can stand the pain any longer.

* I was the first person to try Kangaroo care. The nurses were just great when they saw how content the baby was.

* I'm glad the peer counselor talked me into breastfeeding. I really like it.

- He told me to wean by 12 months so my baby doesn't get tooth decay. That doesn't sound right.

- He won't take my breast! Maybe he just doesn't like me.

- Tim was great when his mother started getting on my case about still nursing Christine. He knew all the right things to say.

- I wish I had listened when my Lamaze teacher said that epidurals don't always work. Mine didn't, and it left me with a terrible backache.

- My boss keeps pressuring me to come back to work, but I don't want to leave my baby.

- I nursed my first baby and really liked it. With my second baby, I was going back to work soon and decided it wasn't worth starting if I couldn't continue.

- I hated weaning Katie when I went back to work. She just cried and cried for my breast for weeks after.

- I thought this hospital had 24-hour rooming-in, but the nurses kept pressuring me to take the baby back to the nursery.

- I'm having a scheduled cesarean because I didn't dilate at all with my first baby. My doctor says I can't give birth naturally.

- This baby is so different from my others. She's so sweet and good-natured!

- The new lactation consultant we hired is really nice. She spent a lot of time with me showing how to get reluctant babies to the breast.

- These new residents are really green. One told me that she'd never seen Kangaroo Care before. We've been doing it for years.

- You're saying to nurse whenever he wants. Won't that spoil him?

- I knew that we both needed treatment for thrush, but the doctor refused to treat the baby because her mouth wasn't white.

- My husband just got laid off and wants me to go to work and he'll take care of the kids. He doesn't even hold the baby when he's home now, and just yells at the others.

- Steve wants to have another baby. I'm not sure, because Tammy still nurses a lot and really seems to need it.

continues

continued

* During the custody hearing, he insisted on unsupervised overnight visits because he says it's time for Joey to wean anyway.

* I can't stand her crying one more minute! She screams constantly.

* I don't know how I'm going to tell my mom that Sara has Down syndrome. She warned me about having a baby when I'm so old.

* Those La Leche League Leaders are just fanatics and want you to keep nursing until the baby is in school.

* That WIC person told me how to eat better, and it made a big difference in how I feel.

* I had no idea that breastfeeding was so good for *me*. I knew it was good for the baby.

* If I go to a support group, I'm afraid that I'll be pushed into nursing longer than I want.

* I couldn't tell him I was still nursing Robbie. He thinks I followed his advice and weaned Robbie a long time ago.

* When I flew home from Atlanta, I had to sit next to a mother who was bottle-feeding her baby. She wasn't tuned into him, and he cried a lot. I'd forgotten how different bottle-feeding is.

* The things she suggested for my engorgement worked well. I'm glad I called.

* I never thought I could breastfeed twins when I had so much trouble with the first one. Getting off to a good start helped a lot!

* It seems that I'm the only one in this clinic that even cares whether the mothers breastfeed. The others couldn't care less.

* I'm not sure I can teach breastfeeding. I didn't nurse my children because it wasn't the thing to do when they were born.

* I heard such bad things about WIC, but you people are really helpful. I wish I'd come sooner.

* He finally nursed for the first time yesterday!

* They are planning to do the heart surgery next week if he gains enough weight. He looks so fragile to me.

* It was so hard to go home and leave her in the Intensive Care Nursery.

* Those night nurses can't seem to understand that the babies do better when they stay in the rooms with their mothers.

* I would never go to that hospital! They make you pay for your own formula.

* Breastfeeding is all right, as long as it's done in private. Those mothers who "flop it out" in the mall are disgusting.

* Bill's mother breastfed all her kids for more than a year, even when it wasn't popular. She's been so supportive of my nursing.

* How in the world will we manage to find 18 hours for training everyone in breast-feeding? We're already short-staffed and pressed for time.

* That old nursing supervisor finally retired. Now we can stop ordering those awful latex nipple shields for our patients.

* Harry really wants me to nurse, but last time it hurt so bad that I'm afraid to even try. I don't think I can make enough milk anyway.

* What is wrong with giving newborns some glucose water? These babies might dehydrate waiting for their mothers' milk to come in.

* I have to teach the next inservice on breastfeeding. I don't know why we bother . . . the clinic mothers aren't interested anyway.

* The new health director wants more emphasis put on breastfeeding. It's about time someone recognized how important it is!

* I got to meet the speaker at lunch, and found out she had trouble nursing her first baby too. I had no idea that these *experts* had real practical experiences as well as their fancy theories.

* She's so cute when she nurses now . . . she pats my breast and smiles up at me.

* I've been teaching breastfeeding for 10 years, and now you say I've been teaching all the wrong things!

* The inservice went better than I thought it would. I didn't realize so many people wanted to learn more about breastfeeding.

* That new baby "superstore" down the street from me sells the same pumps for wholesale prices, and then tells its customers that I'll provide free phone help.

* She rented the pump from the drugstore, then calls me every Friday night when she has questions.

continues

continued

- My baby nurses at least twice at night, and my husband wants to train him to sleep all night, even if it means letting him cry it out.

- I was pumping enough milk for the baby until that setback last week. Now I can hardly get anything, even with the double setup.

- I'm afraid to touch her. The nurses seem so much more competent than I am.

- Emily's mother rarely comes to see her. She sends in her milk but won't come herself, even when we encourage her.

- I don't agree with 24-hour rooming-in. The mothers need their sleep, and I'm going to help them get it.

- They didn't consult *me* when they thought up this new charting scheme. I don't see what was wrong with the old one.

- If we tell the mothers about all the benefits of breastfeeding and then they can't make enough milk, where does that leave them?

- What makes you think you're the expert in breastfeeding here? I've nursed five kids when it wasn't popular. You don't even have one.

- Breastfeeding is only beneficial in third world countries. We don't have problems with diarrhea here.

- I don't want to leave my baby in the church nursery. When I do, she comes back screaming. But I don't want to take her into the church either.

- My mother-in-law wants to keep the baby overnight while we get away for a weekend. Wayne thinks it's a great idea. I'm not sure I trust her . . . she doesn't think I should be breastfeeding.

- I think I'm pregnant again. I wanted to wait longer between babies, but I'm not getting any younger either. Now my nipples are so sore I can't stand nursing.

- I'm supposed to be the breastfeeding coordinator in this department, but ever since Julie took that course she thinks she knows it all.

- My baby gets an ear infection every time I try and give him formula. My doctor says the formula can't possibly cause ear infections, but my sister said it could be an allergy to cow's milk.

* If you think a baby has a short frenulum and refer the parents directly to a dentist, you can forget about getting any more referrals from my office.

* I can't confront the neonatalogist even though I know he's wrong about water bottles for full-termers. I guess the bottles won't hurt the babies too much.

* Just as I think I've got a pregnant mom convinced to try breastfeeding, she sees that one doctor who tells her formula is just as good.

* Can you believe that new doctor? She won't let us give any formula discharge packs to her breastfeeding patients.

* We don't have any breastfeeding supplies in our hospital, and the nearest rental station is 50 miles away.

* If we leave the baby and mother together after delivery, we won't be able to do the admission newborn assessments on time. Then the state will get on our case.

* The state inspector said we should have a lactation consultant. If that is what they want us to do, they should also be providing training.

* If we tell mothers about all the risks of formula, they might feel guilty if they have to use it.

* After I took that lactation course, I just could't stand working with bottle-feeding mothers anymore because of what I learned about formula.

* We do a good job here, then the mothers are sent home where their families don't want them to breastfeed. Why do we even bother?

* Ever since we started using the new breastfeeding policies, our rates have doubled!

* I'm afraid to try cup-feeding. What if the baby chokes?

* These junky pumps, which don't work, really burn me up. You spend lots of money and just get pain and no milk for it. Why do they keep making them?

* This electric pump is really slick. I was afraid of using it at first because I thought it would hurt. My girlfriend said her pump made her nipples sore.

* They finally put in a pump for the staff to use, but it's way down in the employee lounge, and I can't be away from my station long enough to use it.

* No matter what I say to pregnant women, they've already made up their minds about feeding before they even get to see me.

FEELING WORD VOCABULARY

Intense (+)	Strong (+)	Moderate (+)	Mild (+)	Mild (−)	Moderate (−)	Strong (−)	Intense (−)
loved	enhanced	liked	friendly	unpopular	suspicious	disgusted	hate
adored	ardor	cared-for	regarded		envious	resentful	unloved
idolized	infatuated	esteemed	benevolent		enmity	bitter	abhor
	tender	affectionate			aversion	detested	loathed
		fond				fed-up	despised
alive	vibrant	excited	wide-awake	listless	dejected	frustrated	angry
	independent	patient	at-ease	moody	unhappy	sad	hurt
	capable	strong	relaxed	lethargic	bored	depressed	miserable
	happy	good	comfortable	gloomy	bad	sick	pain
	great	inspired	content	dismal	forlorn	disconsolate	lonely
	proud	strong	amazed	discontented	disappointed	dissatisfied	cynical
	gratified	amused	alert	tired	wearied	fatigued	exhausted
			sensitive				
wanted	worthy	secure	sure	indifferent	torn-up	worn-out	worthless
lustful	passionate	yearning	attractive	unsure	inadequate	useless	impotent
worthy	admired	popular	approved	impatient	ineffectual	weak	futile
pity	sympathetic	peaceful	untroubled	dependent	helpless	hopeless	abandoned
respected	important	appealing	graceful	unimportant	resigned	forlorn	estranged
empathy	concerned	determined		regretful	apathetic	rejected	degraded
awed	appreciated			bashful	shamed	guilty	humiliated
	consoled			self-conscious	shy	embarrassed	alienated
					uncomfortable	inhibited	
elation	delighted	pleased	turned-on	puzzled	baffled	bewildered	shocked
enthusiastic	eager	excited	warm	edgy	confused	frightened	panicky
zealous	optimistic	interested	amused	upset	nervous	anxious	trapped
	joyful	jolly		reluctant	tempted	dismayed	horrified
	courage	relieved		timid	tense	apprehensive	afraid
	hopeful	glad		mixed-up	worried	dreadful	scared
					perplexed	disturbed	terrified
					troubled		threatened
courageous	valiant	adventurous	daring	sullen	disdainful	antagonistic	infuriated
	brave	peaceful	comfortable	provoked	contemptuous	vengeful	furious
	brilliant	intelligent	smart		alarmed	indignant	
					annoyed	mad	
					provoked		

Adapted from La Leche League's *Human Relations Workbook, 1982.*

SOLVING THE PUZZLE: INFANT ILLNESS/BREASTFEEDING CARE PLAN EXERCISE[4]

GOAL

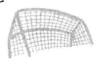

To develop comprehensive breastfeeding management plans for specific infant illnesses and/or conditions using a team approach

BEST AUDIENCE

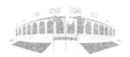

Health-care professionals and lactation management students. For this game, the instructor must have a deep and thorough knowledge of clinical breastfeeding management.

TIME REQUIRED

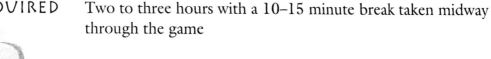

Two to three hours with a 10–15 minute break taken midway through the game

HOW TO PLAY

To set up the game, prepare case histories of 10–12 breastfeeding children who each have a different medical and/or breastfeeding problem. The case description should include age, weight, pertinent social/family history, and circumstances. All mothers of the children have stated their goal is to breastfeed exclusively for about six months and continue breastfeeding for at least a year. Some babies should be past the newborn period. Assume that the medical/professional political climate in these cases is friendly to and supportive of breastfeeding—this is not an exercise in playing politics.

Have ready several pads of flip chart (newsprint) paper, tape, and plenty of colored markers—black plus seven other colors will do. Prepare four to six name tags for the other *professional team members*—physicians, dietitians, social workers, La Leche League Leaders, physical/occupational therapists, and nurses.

[4]**Source:** This game was originally developed for the *Lactation Consultant Exam Preparation Course* taught through Lact-Ed, Inc.

Encourage the students to bring textbooks and reference materials to class. I always provide a classroom library of pertinent texts and references.

Part One:

Divide the group so that two to four students work on each case. Ask each person to work with a person they have never worked with before. No one should work alone. If necessary, three students can work on two cases to alleviate this problem. The cases can be assigned by the faculty or chosen by the groups.

Allow about an hour for students to research each illness/clinical situation in textbooks, the classroom library, and so on. (Alternative: Assign the cases at the close of a clinical teaching day. The students' *homework* is to research the cases. Resume the exercise on a subsequent instructional day.)

After researching the clinical problem, each team will develop a *specific* and *detailed* care plan that includes goals; immediate (on-site) interventions with rationales; and short- and long-term follow-up plans. The goal of the plan is to establish or restore breastfeeding in the context of the infant's illness or condition and create/reinforce behaviors to encourage extended breastfeeding.

As the LC developing the plan, assume you are responsible for coordinating the lactation care of this baby and mother. Your assessments will be supported, and your recommendations will be followed. Focus on the *specific* baby and mother in each case history. Once again, assume the political and clinical climate is knowledgeable and supportive of breastfeeding.

Focus on establishing or re-establishing breastfeeding first. Be specific and include the pertinent information. For example, if breast pumping is a suggested strategy, include the following information:

* Specific equipment

* Reason for choosing a specific device

* How often and how long to use the device

* Milk storage details

* How the milk will be fed to the baby

* Rationale for why this particular feeding method was chosen

* How direct breastfeeding will eventually be initiated/resumed

After effective feeding is established, then address other physical or social issues that will affect breastfeeding in the long term. If you want further evaluation or treatment by another care provider, be sure to include that in the plan.

If more than one strategy could be considered, describe *Plan A* with rationale and expected outcomes. In addition, include a *Plan B* if results of Plan A are unsatisfactory and also include how that decision will be made.

Each team should write out its care plan(s) onto the large papers using *black* markers and post these care plans around the room on the walls. Ask them to leave space for further comments. After all the care plans are posted, regather the group.

Part Two:

Next, the group will take on the roles of other health care providers to *add to* the lactation care plans. Redivide the group into six teams, each assuming the role of one of the following health care providers—physicians, nurses, physical and occupational therapists, dietitians, social workers, and La Leche League Leaders. Give each *team* a different color of marker and the prepared *profession* name tags you created earlier. Instructors (faculty) will use a different color of marker from all the other groups.

Have each group circulate among all posted care plans and add any further comments from their profession's perspective to each of the specific cases. If no professional role is appropriate for a team, they should sign *no role for XXX*. Groups should write these comments and any other recommendations directly on the large papers.

Instructors (faculty) also circulate to all of the posted plans, and using a different color marker from all the other groups, add any necessary corrections (be gentle with your corrections, please), suggestions, information, questions on why a certain strategy was chosen, references, praise for especially astute thinking, and so on.

Conclusion/wrap-up:

Some groups will want to copy down the detailed information on all of the care plans. I gently discourage this because every baby is different. It is more productive in the long run to encourage students to take their own notes on the *process* used in this exercise and how they approached each infant situation.

Review each of the cases and discuss the pertinent lactation issues for each infant condition. Emphasize the importance of critical thinking, individualized care strategies, and the team approach. When I conduct this game, I bring research articles or citations, point out relevant chapters in professional texts, and encourage discussion of possible alternative therapies or approaches.

Teaching tip: Do not rush this exercise. The careful analysis of each individual baby and family reinforces the concept that the baby does not exist in isolation and that "cookbook" remedies are only the beginning of an approach to any given baby. The best results from this game occur when sufficient time is allocated to explore each illness/condition in depth.

Teaching tip: A few cases are included as models. Use these cases, and/or write up your own clients (without using their real names.)

SAMPLE CASE HISTORIES

Preterm Twins—One Has Thrush

José and Maria were born at 36 weeks gestation, weighing 6 lbs, 11 oz (3 kg) and 5 lbs, 2 oz (2.4 kg) respectively. Juanita requested a home visit at six weeks post birth. She has been using a breast pump for six weeks; her nipples are tender and slightly red. José nurses exclusively at breast. Maria gets pumped milk via bottle. Juanita is still having a hard time accepting twins. Juanita says her goal is to "keep nursing both; for Maria to gain weight faster; use my milk for both; and keep my sanity. I halfway want Maria to have bottles because it's too hard to handle both at breast."

José now weighs 9 lbs, 14 oz (4.5 kg) in a t-shirt and dry diaper—a gain of nearly 3 lbs (1.4 kg) in six weeks. Although his skin tone is slightly yellow, he is otherwise healthy and alert. At breast, José's nursing is somewhat disorganized but of appropriate duration with self-detachment. His tongue is coated with thick white plaques, and he has a red rash in the anal/diaper area.

Maria's weight was 7 lbs, 6½ oz (3.5 kg)—a gain of 3 lbs (1.4 kg) from her low weight of four lbs (2 kg). Juanita's live-in nanny had fed Maria about 2 oz (60 ml) of pumped milk via bottle shortly before the LC arrived. When Maria awoke about 90 minutes later, Juanita wanted to try finger-feeding instead of putting Maria to breast. Maria latched on shallowly with moderately disorganized tongue peristalsis and posterior humping. She took about ½ ounce (15 ml) with the finger-feeding device. Juanita did not attempt to put Maria to breast during this visit.

Cystic Fibrosis

Sophia is four months old. At two weeks of age, she was exclusively breastfed but is now failing to thrive. Her mother, Miranda, was told that breastfeeding was the problem and was instructed to wean and feed Sophia with a cow's milk-based infant formula. However, Sophia's weight gain did not improve, and she began to have repeated bouts of bronchitis and pneumonia, including one that required hospitalization. Shortly thereafter, Sophia was diagnosed with Cystic Fibrosis (CF) and is currently being fed a predigested infant formula.

Miranda has many questions about Sophia's nutrition and has considered buying goat's milk for her. At one point, Miranda rented an electric breast pump and briefly attempted to bring her milk back in but was quickly discouraged by a health care provider who said breastmilk was not recommended for babies with CF. Miranda says that Sophia still seeks her breast at bedtime.

Miranda has two other children ages three and five and provides day care to several other preschool-age children. She wants to give her baby the best nutrition possible and include breastfeeding in her parenting goals.

Birth Injury—Poor Suck

Claire was born at 41 weeks gestation, weighing 9 lbs, 8 oz (4.3 kg). Her mother, Rachelle, had elevated blood pressure and swollen ankles and fingers in the last week of her pregnancy.

Rachelle's extended family came to town about a week ago for a family reunion. On the same day that Rachelle's labor began, her mother suddenly developed chest pains and was rushed to a cardiac care unit in the same hospital. Unbeknownst to Rachelle, her mother died from a ruptured aortic aneurysm during Rachelle's labor. Rachelle's doctor slowed her labor so that the baby would be born on a different day than the day of her mother's death. The labor was over 12 hours long. An epidural was administered when Rachelle was 8 cm dilated, and delivery was assisted with a vacuum extractor. Clarie's APGAR scores were seven and nine.

Clarie is now four days old and cannot latch on and feed effectively. Her skin is slightly yellow, although she has had four profuse stools and four soaking wet diapers in the past 18 hours. Her weight today is 9 lbs, 4 oz (4.2 kg)—the same as her discharge weight on Day two. She has a pronounced preference to turn her head to the right, with marked facial asymmetry. Rachelle has been pumping every two to three hours with a hospital-grade electric pump and giving the milk to Claire with a dropper. Rachelle's right nipple is scabbed, her left one is normal, and both breasts are full of milk with mild edema around the areola. At Rachelle's breast, Claire attempts to latch, but she either takes a few swallows and screams or falls asleep.

Failure to Thrive

Amanda is 34 years old with a history of thyroid irregularities and mild asthma. Her other children, ages three and five, were breastfed more than a year each, and The three year old has eczema, asthma, and has had chronic otitis media. Amanda gave birth to Kyle by scheduled cesarean delivery with vacuum assistance. Kyle first nursed about three hours after birth; Amanda described it as "poor." Onset of a copious milk supply occurred on day 4. Kyle had lost more than 10 percent of his birthweight by 48 hours post partum, so supplements of expressed breastmilk were started on day two using a feeding tube placed along Amanda's finger and/or a small cup. Amanda reports pacifier use of "a half hour or so" each day. She says Kyle has a functional heart murmur and a ventricular septal defect.

continues

continued

At four weeks old, Kyle is thin and sleepy with a rash on his cheeks. Overall muscle tone is lower than expected for 4½ weeks of age. Oral structures are normal; oral motor tone is within normal limits. Tongue peristalsis is inconsistent with posterior humping. Kyle's weight was 8 lbs, 9 oz (3.9 kg) at a pediatric visit two days ago. At breast, Kyle signals poorly, yet Amanda quickly responds to his subtle cues. Kyle achieved an acceptable latch in the cradle position on the right breast, but quickly dozed off. When Amanda's milk let-down, he sustained two to three minutes of moderately organized sucking. Total feed length was about five to six minutes. Amanda easily pumped 2.5 oz (71 ml) from each breast (a total of 5 oz [150 ml]), which she fed to Kyle using a feeding tube device. He took the full 5 oz (150 ml), exhibited organized sucking patterns during the entire duration, and then self-detached in obvious satiation. Amanda's stated goal is to have Kyle nursing effectively at breast.

Birth Injury

Abbey is five days old, sleepy with slightly yellow skin. There is a 1-inch (2.54 cm) diameter cephalhematoma on the left side of her crown. Her suck is somewhat gentle with inconsistent tongue humping and cheek puckering. At breast, Abbey latches on easily and sustains organized patterns for about five to eight minutes, then shows some disorganized sucking bursts, then self-detaches. She cues to eat again within about 15–20 minutes. She is more organized when her left shoulder is higher than the right. During labor, her mother, Dolores, received IV narcotics and epidural anesthesia. Birth was assisted with a vacuum extractor. Dolores says her milk supply is abundant without edema or engorgement, and her nipples are comfortable. Abbey has six or more wet diapers per day and more than three yellow stools. Pacifier use is sporadic.

Tongue-tie

Peter is 12 days old but weighs only 9 oz (270 g) above his birth weight of 6 lbs, 13 oz (3.1 kg). His mother, Nancy, has a positive history for "many allergies." Her labor was induced at 35 weeks because of toxemia. Nancy received two epidurals in addition to IV narcotics and a tranquilizer during labor. She pushed for 2½ hours before birth was assisted with a vacuum extractor. Nancy stopped breastfeeding from days four through eight because of bruised and "bloody slashes" on her nipples. Peter now attempts to breastfeed about every two hours for about 10 minutes on each breast or on one breast for 20 minutes. He is also receiving supplemental formula by bottle. Nancy's milk supply is low, and she does not feel a let-down reflex. Both nipple tips have scabs in the center; and both areolae are pink and slightly inflamed. She expressed some milk from each breast a few minutes ago.

Peter's lingual frenulum is short and tight, but attached normally to the tongue and lower gum ridge. There are white patches on his tongue. Tongue peristalsis is poor and disorganized with significant retraction and posterior humping. Palate shape is normal. Peter attempts to latch but does not take the breast deeply into his mouth. Once latched, he enjoys being at breast, but is unable to effectively take milk for more than a few moments during a 10–15 minute feeding. Even with a disorganized suck, Peter can manage to take in about 1.5 oz (45 ml) of formula from a bottle using a slow-flow style teat (nipple). Nancy says her goals are to breastfeed exclusively for six months and then continue breastfeeding for 18 months. No one has helped her with breastfeeding since she left the hospital. Her family life is chaotic due to a recent move and her husband's work schedule.

Nursing Strike

Jillian's baby, Mary, is 13 months old. Mary suddenly refused to nurse three days ago, at the start of her fourth ear infection in the past three months. Jillian has been pumping her milk and giving it to Mary in a spouted cup. Mary enthusiastically drinks the milk but refuses to come to breast. Mary cannot tolerate cow's milk formula. Jillian also tried goat's milk without success. Mary will eat rice cereal and some vegetables; however she cannot tolerate most protein-rich foods. At about four weeks old, Jillian started giving Mary a pacifier so that she would sleep in her crib. Jillian is very distressed that Mary refuses to breastfeed.

Hydrocephalus and Tongue-tie

Cameron is 3½ weeks old. Hydrocephalus was diagnosed prebirth, and even with a shunt surgically implanted, his head is very large and heavy. His mother, Katie, thought that the hydrocephalus was affecting his ability to suck, until she realized that his lingual frenulum was short and tight. She has been pumping her milk since he was born, giving it to him with a standard bottle and nipple. Katie strongly desires to nurse Cameron at her breast, as she did with her other four children.

Biting

Andy is 5½ months old and just starting to eat small amounts of family food. His mother Jessica complains that he has begun to bite at the end of nursing sessions, as he is falling asleep at breast. Because he has two teeth, this biting is damaging her nipples. She nursed her other two children for only a few months each and wants to continue nursing Andy at least a year if she can get him to stop biting.

continues

continued

Reflux

William is eight weeks old and is exclusively breastfed. His mother, Kay, is miserable—he only stops crying when she holds him vertically against her chest. He screams as if he is in pain if she puts him down on his back or stomach. He will nap for about 15 minutes when placed on his side, however he sleeps best when Kay is in a reclining chair with William resting semi-prone on her chest. He has gained more than two pounds since his birth and is otherwise normal and healthy. William spits up after nearly every feed and gags when Kay's milk lets down. Kay is intolerant to cow's milk and soy and monitors her own diet very closely to avoid these foods.

Jaundice

Grace is three days old, sleepy, and her skin appears yellow down to her knees. She had one void today and has not yet stooled since she passed meconium on the first day post birth. Her mother, Julia, has tried to get her to latch—without success. Julia's breasts are full and hard.

Thrush

Anita has three-week-old identical twins, Cara and Carlie. Their sibling, Emily, is 23 months old. Anita's nipples are sore, and she has scabs on the tips of both nipples. Cara has been so "slow" at breast that Anita decided to put Cara on a bottle. Anita's breasts now seem less full. Inside Cara's mouth are white patches on her tongue, gums, and buccal mucosa.

Allergy

Tamika is not sure that her milk is good, because her baby is very gassy and fussy in the evenings. She gives one-month-old Kano two bottles of cow's milk-based formula every day. Kano is gaining 2 oz (60 g) per day, is voiding well, but is having difficulty passing his stool. He goes to breast easily, but after a few minutes, he stiffens, arches away, and cries. Tamika is also worried because he had an ear infection last week and has had a persistent itchy rash on his face.

Cleft Palate

Nicole's baby, Emma, was 7 lbs, 15.8 oz (3.6 kg) at birth. Emma is now three days old and was born with a unilateral cleft of the upper lip. Emma is otherwise healthy. Nicole hopes to breastfeed for at least a year.

Prematurity

Samira delivered baby Hamid at 34 weeks gestation after being on bed rest for six weeks for preterm labor. Four-day-old Hamid weighed 3 lbs, 8 oz (1600 g) at birth, is on room air, and is in an open bed. Samira is beginning to feel some breast fullness, but so far she has been able to pump only a few drops of "clear fluid." She is afraid that she won't be able to make enough milk.

Down Syndrome

Daniel has Down syndrome. He weighed 7 lbs, 4 oz (3.3 kg) at birth and is now nine days old. He has lost more than 1 lb (.5 kg) from birth weight and is having difficulty at breast. Sandra uses meticulous positioning and latch-on techniques but Daniel has difficulty maintaining suction at breast. His tongue keeps hanging out of his mouth. Sandra was told to supplement Daniel, but he vomits whenever she gives him artificial baby milk. Daniel has no signs of cardiac problems. Sandra is having a hard time accepting Daniel's condition, and her husband, Rick, refuses to hold Daniel at all.

Cardiac Disease

Vanessa is two weeks old and has a cardiac defect. She has difficulty sustaining any long periods of activity and is not gaining well despite being bottle-fed several times per day. She vomits most of her cow's milk-based formula but tolerates expressed breastmilk well. The doctor wants to add a calorie booster to all of Vanessa's feedings. Additionally, Vanessa has to be fed in an upright position, because laying flat causes her to have respiratory difficulty from retained fluids. Darleen, Vanessa's mother, has a single attachment kit for an electric breast pump but is using it manually. She desperately wants to breastfeed, and Vanessa enjoys being breastfed.

Feeding Problem Due to Milk Oversupply

Zoe is almost ready to quit breastfeeding because her baby Miles chokes, gasps, and struggles during most breastfeeds. He feeds better in the evening and at night than in the morning and early afternoon. Miles has nearly tripled his birth weight in three months. His stools are profuse and often green, watery, and "explosive." In addition, Zoe complains that her breasts leak milk constantly, and she is uncomfortably full of milk much of the time. Zoe would like breastfeeding to be pleasant and relaxed for both Miles and herself.

JELLY BELLY GAME[5]

GOAL 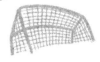	To understand aromatic properties of human milk and protective mechanisms of breastfeeding
BEST AUDIENCE 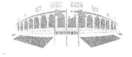	Any
TIME REQUIRED	Five minutes to prepare the room; 5–10 minutes to play
HOW TO PLAY	*Props needed:* Enough JellyBelly™ jellybean candies in assorted flavors so that each participant gets at least two. If possible, purchase the individually wrapped variety. (Note: Other brands don't work as well.)

Distribute at least two JellyBellies to each participant and warn them to *not* eat them yet. Give players the following instructions:

1. Unwrap or select one JellyBelly and get ready to put it in your mouth.

2. Hold your nose. While continuing to hold your nose, place one JellyBelly in your mouth and chew it a few times.

3. Now release your nose and continue chewing.

When the nose is released, the aroma of the candy floods the oral and nasal cavities. Usually the audience exhales a collective, "oooh," when the aroma of the candy is released. Tell them that they can eat the other JellyBellies.

[5]**Source:** I learned this game from Kay Hoover, MEd, IBCLC, who learned it from Julie Menella, PhD.

This activity suggests how breastmilk sprays from the nipple into the posterior oropharynx, coating the nasal turbinates. Aromas that the baby has smelled in amniotic fluid for several months are also in the milk, which helps the baby become further acculturated to family foods. Furthermore, the fine sprays of milk coat the mucus membranes in the baby's mouth, nose, and throat, enabling the white cells and other immunoactors to attack surface-borne pathogens.

LATCH-ON GROUP GAME

GOAL

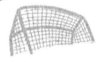

To teach effective and comfortable latch-on and positioning at breast, which is a basic skill for new mothers

BEST AUDIENCE

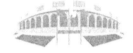

Any; each person needs a newborn-size doll. If enough dolls are not available for everyone, the minimum number needed is one doll per three students.

TIME REQUIRED

Fifteen minutes per "role," 45–60 minutes total

HOW TO PLAY

The instructor demonstrates good technique with a doll and breast model in front of the entire group by going through the entire positioning and latch process: position the baby, support the breast, latch-on, relax, and continue nursing. Demonstrate at least two positions at breast (cradle, clutch, preemie, or lying down).

Parent groups: Couples work together with Dad being the first "mom." Or, you can place the men together in groups of three and the women in separate groups of three.

Professionals: Divide them into groups of three. This game works best when the instructor divides the group (for example, with with stickers as they enter the room) in a way that breaks up companions. Participants need to feel like strangers in their groups.

This game is played several times so that everyone plays all roles—mom, teacher/nurse, and observer/dad. Mom starts with the doll. Teacher helps mom get her baby to nurse. Observer watches what happens but does not interfere. The baby should be at the breast within two to three minutes.

After the first round, ask one participant at a time how it felt to play their assigned role. Then ask the other two how it felt to them and what they observed. Repeat with players changing roles *and* groups. (For example, have all the "moms" move to another group and assume a different role.) Circulate and jot down comments that you later share with the groups. Natural leaders will emerge within groups. Personal breastfeeding stories should be encouraged. This breaks the ice wonderfully in professional inservices.

Note: This game is particularly effective for those who have never personally nursed a baby. Even in groups of experienced people, something new can be learned. *Take your time* and do not rush this game, because you are teaching a fundamental skill. Comments, such as "We don't have time," will arise, which will lead into discussions about how policies should support biology. Breastfeeding assistance must proceed at the baby's pace.

LIFECYCLE OF THE MOTHER-BABY BREASTFEEDING DYAD[6]

GOAL

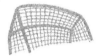

To correlate the baby's developmental stages (time continuum) with diverse aspects of maternal development, infant development, and the developing mother-baby breastfeeding relationship. This game helps students grasp the interrelated and interwoven matrix of maternal-infant developmental stages.

Note: After many failed attempts at having students research each aspect of infant or maternal development separately, the structure for this game emerged. I have not yet found a published source where maternal and infant development are cross-correlated, yet lactation counselors are expected to keep these aspects in mind when helping an individual dyad or when designing a breastfeeding care and promotion program.

BEST AUDIENCE

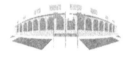

Health care professionals and lactation-management students. For this game, the instructor must have a deep and thorough knowledge of the subject matter in order to answer questions that may be posed by students.

TIME REQUIRED

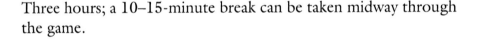

Three hours; a 10–15-minute break can be taken midway through the game.

HOW TO PLAY

The preparation for this game is crucial, challenging, and time-consuming.

---

[6] **Source:** This game was originally developed for the *Lactation Consultant Exam Preparation Course* formerly taught through Lact-Ed, Inc.

Setup:

1. You need a backboard large enough to hold 120 pieces of information and yet small enough that students can manipulate, rearrange, and read the individual pieces. The backboard can be a large piece of sturdy fabric or felt that can be hung on a wall, FoamCore™ board that can stand alone, a tabletop display, or some other sturdy backing material. Set up the grid on the backboard by either marking the topic headings directly on the backboard or by using a different color card for the headings. See the chart that follows these instructions for how the finished layout should appear.

2. Information cards should be small enough to hold and rearrange, yet large enough to be readable, and should fasten onto the backboard. I used computer software designed to create business cards to create my game cards, using a different color cardboard stock for each horizontal continuum. I laminated each card and placed a piece of Velcro™ on the back. I arranged the matching pieces of Velcro™ on the backboard. Other methods of sticking the cards to the backboard can be used, as long as the cards can be rearranged.

3. If you regularly teach large groups, prepare multiple sets of backboards and cards. One backboard and set of information cards can be used by up to 10 people.

Part 1:

4. Divide the class into groups so that 5–10 people work together with one set of materials.

5. Students should sort the cards into categories first and then arrange each category (continuum) in chronological order according to the developmental stage. Students may use any references available to help in this task, *except* the prepared chart for this exercise.

6. After each category is arranged in order, place the cards on the backboard. Each age/stage can have only one card, but one card may span more than one age/stage. In that case, place the card at the younger (lower) end of the range that it spans.

7. If multiple groups are doing this exercise, have them circulate to other teams' backboards and compare results and then return to their own boards and make any changes they feel necessary. Also allow students to compare their results to the printed chart. Allow 10–15 minutes for discussion, clarification of the various categories of development, etc.

Part 2:

8. Redivide the class into 12 groups to represent the 12 ages/stages on the chart. The cards were placed on the grid horizontally but will be removed vertically. Collect all the cards that apply to one developmental age and give them to one group. Repeat until each group has a set of cards pertinent to a specific developmental age/stage. (If the class is small, give each group two ages/stages.)

9. Each group will examine the developmental milestones, events, and tasks of that particular age and develop a *brief core concept* or *theme* for that age. The core concept should be expressed in a sentence, short paragraph, poem, song, or other mode of expression, which will communicate the unique aspects of that age/stage.

LIFECYCLE OF THE BREASTFEEDING MOTHER-BABY DYAD

10 Aspects of Maternal and Infant Development Cross-Correlated to 12 Developmental Stages

Continuum	General Principles	Pre-conception	Prenatal	Labor & Birth	Prematurity
Physical growth; growth curves	Occurs in spurts; height and weight spurts alternate	Heredity and environment play a strong role. Optimal intrauterine environment begins in the woman's own infancy.	25% of brain growth	Avg. size 7–8 lbs, 21" long	< 37 wks gestation, <2500 gm in weight.
Psychomotor development; behavioral state; sleep patterns	The infant is immature in nearly every bodily system; development emerges along a biologically-determined timetable.	Adult sleep patterns vary; myths of need for uninterrupted sleep are common.	Able to suck at 32 wks; sleep cycles and movement patterns may be hints of later behavior	Rooting, tongue extrusion reflexes present at birth. Quiet alert state starts shortly after birth; infant able to self-attach at breast in about an hour.	Poor coordination overall; weak; tires easily. Kangaroo Care fosters deep, restful sleep.

10. Finally, have each team (in chronological order) present the core concept of that developmental stage to the large group.

11. Allow time for discussion and synthesis of how the maternal and infant developmental tasks interact with one another.

1–2 Days	3–14 Days	15–28 Days	1–3 months	4–6 months	7–12 months	Over 12 months
0–7% wt loss tolerated	Regain birth weight by 7–10 days; growth spurt at about 14 days	½ – 2 oz/day wt gain; avg. .75 oz	Head circumference larger than artificially fed	Double birth weight by 6 months; 50% of brain growth complete. Artificially fed are heavier per length.	Triple birth weight by 12 months; 67% of brain growth complete.	Artificially fed are fatter through 18 months; larger difference in males
Palmar grasp; stepping; raises head; activity ceases when hearing sounds, stares; follows to midline.	Tonic neck reflex; roots and sucks well. Sleeps best when close to mother	Continued need for night feeds; co-sleeping fosters deep sleep.	Integration of reflexes, raises head longer and higher from prone; turns head toward noise, eyes follow past midline, brief holding of hands, head sags in sitting, flexes legs	Parachute reaction; rests on forearms with head high; turns head toward bell; consistent regard; engages in fingerplay; corraling with both hands; sits with body erect, head supported.	Visual pursuit of dropped objects; shifts eyes from object to person; hands versatile and active; pincer grasp; throws; crawls, pulls up and may walk; sits unsupported; pivots.	Walks with support, runs; grasps implements, self-feeds.

continues

continued

Continuum	General Principles	Pre-conception	Prenatal	Labor & Birth	Prematurity
Sensorimotor	Uses senses, motor skills & reflexes to explore; develops schemas to deal with information and experiences: reasoning thought, perception		Mouth is primary; body is secondary organ of exploration with unknown start point.		
Psychosocial (attachment)	Trust/ integrity develops as mother appropriately and consistently responds to baby's cues. If she responds, the next stage is easier for baby; if she does not, the baby must struggle with both simultaneously	Early childhood experiences affect later behavior	Trust vs. mistrust. Prebirth bonding research suggests that babies are sentient before birth.	Doula research suggests that mothers care for their babies as they were cared for during labor and birth.	Developmental, humanized care for preterms, including Kangaroo Care, fosters optimal attachment and bonding

1–2 Days	3–14 Days	15–28 Days	1–3 months	4–6 months	7–12 months	Over 12 months
Mostly reflexive behavior; sucking, swallowing, grasping, rooting.	Reflexes start to be replaced by voluntary activity	Recognizes familiar faces and objects; anticipates feeds. Beginning of primary circular reactions	Mouth and hands are primary organs of exploration; body is secondary	Searches for objects that have fallen, tolerates some frustration; some delayed gratification	Mouth, hands and body are equally important. Stranger anxiety, individuation. Attracts attention deliberately.	Object permanence, able to think before taking action; individuation continues.
Trust vs. mistrust continues; separation causes biological and psychological stress to both	Trust continues to develop with responsive mothering	Trust continues to develop with responsive mothering	Continued presence of mother helps forge secure attachment	Friendly, outgoing behavior if maternal attachment is secure	Stranger anxiety peaks; knows mother is different from all others in the world.	Autonomy vs. shame.

continues

continued

Continuum	General Principles	Pre-conception	Prenatal	Labor & Birth	Prematurity
Adaptive-Social	Way of actively seeking attention changes as baby develops		Knows mother	Knows mother	Knows mother
Breastfeeding & feeding behaviors	Breastfeeding is the biological norm for the baby	A mother's first breastfeeding experience affects her behavior in subsequent pregnancies	Laying skill foundation for oral feeds; swallow amniotic fluids; sucking releases gut hormones.	Baby is active participant in feeding process; frequent cues to feed; can self-attach. Variable frequency and duration.	Tires easily; feeds may be shorter; easier to breastfeed than bottle-feed at same developmental age; sleeps to save energy.

1–2 Days	3–14 Days	15–28 Days	1–3 months	4–6 months	7–12 months	Over 12 months
Mews, tearless crying, effectively communicates hunger, differentiable cries.	Attachment parenting reduces need to cry	Eye-to-eye contact especially important; focal distance is 8–10"	Babbles, coos, blows bubbles, obvious social smiling	Coos, converses, talks to toys or self. Rapid change from tears to smiles, laughs aloud, initiates contact with smiling, obvious recognition of siblings and father.	Vocalizes "dada" & "mama," responds to simple questions; waves bye-bye, adjusts to simple commands, smiles at mirror image.	Responds to commands by taking action, offers others objects.
Variable frequency and duration, hands to face = hunger cue. Exclusive colostrum feeds; easy to coordinate suck-swallow-breathe	Increasing milk volume; feeds total at least 140 minutes per day; baby sets own patterns; mother increasingly able to read cues; exclusive breastfeeding.	Cluster feeds, at least 140 minutes per 24-hour day; exclusive breastfeeding. Patterns may begin to emerge. Exclusive breastfeeding.	More predictability, baby truly drives galactopoiesis. By 3 months, baby will stop feed to attend to stimulus. Exclusive breastfeeding	Baby more efficient at milk transfer; easily distracted especially during day; more frequent night nursing. Exclusive breastfeeding.	Lifts up mother's shirt, acrobatics. Spontaneous desire for family foods. Allergic babies may delay intake of solids. Substantial breastfeeding	May have special word for breastfeeding; may want to stand up, asks to feed. Breastfeeding is still a substantial source of nutrients, calories, and immune protection.

continues

continued

Continuum	General Principles	Pre-conception	Prenatal	Labor & Birth	Prematurity
Biosexual, changes; maternal fertility	Biosexual events (or lack thereof) are a large part of women's health issues and have lifelong and life-changing impact.	Women's reproductive health begins in her own childhood and youth	Onset of pregnancy changes perception of sexuality; broadens it	Experience colors all aspects of sexuality; premiere biosexual event.	Sense of failure to achieve completion of premier event
Maternal role acquisition	Mothering is one unique aspect of female development	Observations of family; friends, fantasizing about motherhood; planning to get pregnant.	Validation ("I'm pregnant"); fetal embodiment (baby's inside) heightened by quickening; fetal distinction (baby's coming out). Changes by trimester. Making lifestyle changes to protect baby (giving up, letting go).	Bridge from "baby is in" to "baby is out," completes process of fetal distinction; role transition; opening up to baby after engrossment with physical events of labor.	May hold back from attachment for fear of baby's death or fragility; may blame self. Grieving.

1–2 Days	3–14 Days	15–28 Days	1–3 months	4–6 months	7–12 months	Over 12 months
Immersed in physical aspects of birth & postpartum; transition from pregnancy to external gestation	Lactational Amennorrhea Method of family planning (LAM): no bleeds, exclusive breastfeeding, baby under 6 months = <1% risk of conception	Possible desire to return to intercourse or wants to avoid it	Lactation as biosexual function more fully realized by mother by this time. Feels more comfortable with breasts as more than and other than sexual organs.	Possible return to fertility.	Possible desire for another baby. Possible return to fertility.	14.2 months is average ending of lactational amennorrhea.
Grieving lost expectations; taking-in; "should do" or "must do;" fantasy of mother-hood and baby starts being replaced by reality.	Taking hold; taking on; "should do, must do," may do, I do. Fantasy is replaced by reality. Grieving lost expectations.	Learning coping skills, "honeymoon is over."	Settling in; increase in self-confidence and ability to produce milk and nurture baby. Mothers "may do," testing theories against reality. Ambivalence about returning to outside work. Firmly attached to baby.	Increased pride in self and baby. Joy and delight.	Most are at "I do" stage. May doubt self when baby is in shy (stranger anx-iety) stage. Continued joy and delight in baby.	Confident in abilities.

continues

continued

Continuum	General Principles	Pre-conception	Prenatal	Labor & Birth	Prematurity
Maternal Physical changes	Pregnancy, birth and lactation cause profound metabolic and physiologic changes	Childhood diet and health may affect development of breast structures and reproductive capacity	Breast changes; growing fetus; requires lifestyle changes; heightened body awareness (captive audience).	Most profound normal physical event she may ever experience.	Preterm birth may be difficult physically
Lactogenesis & galactopoiesis	Women's bodies follow a biological timetable for breast growth and development	Ductal and breast development with menstrual cycles.	Breast development accelerates; Lactogenesis I (colostrum) starts around 4 months gestation and continues.	Placental separation and withdrawal of progesterone signals Lactogenesis II to begin.	Milk composition tailored to baby's developmental age.

1–2 Days	3–14 Days	15–28 Days	1–3 months	4–6 months	7–12 months	Over 12 months
Physical discomfort, healing begins	Transition to lactation "figure," breasts softer after any edema is past.	Gradual weight loss, appetite changes, exhaustion, vaginal dryness, cessation of postpartum bleeding.	Uterine involution complete. Feels good.	Weight loss may continue or plateau. Body utilizes nutrients efficiently during lactation.	Loss of pregnancy-related weight nearly or fully complete	Feels healthy; re-accumulating body stores of nutrients.
Lactogenesis III begins around 30–50 hours post birth with an increase in lactose and fluid volume.	Rapidly increasing milk volume; autocrine control of milk synthesis beginning	By 6 weeks, full lactogenesis complete; endocrine control giving way to autocrine control. Volume stabilizing 15–25% ahead of baby's needs.	No significant changes in milk synthesis; continuing adjustment to baby's needs.	Milk volume stays relatively steady; continuing adjustment to baby's needs.	As baby weans, regression milk has less lactose and fluid volume. Return to colostrum if subsequent pregnancy occurs.	Synthesis continues with consistent removal of milk.

MOCK TRIAL[7]

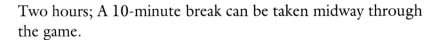

GOAL

To teach/explore legal issues related to breastfeeding and lactation consultant practice

BEST AUDIENCE

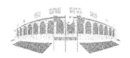

Health care professionals, lactation consultants, and lactation management students. For this game, the instructor must have a deep and thorough knowledge of the subject matter in order to answer questions that may be posed by students.

TIME REQUIRED

Two hours; A 10-minute break can be taken midway through the game.

HOW TO PLAY

Setup:

1. Find a gavel and black robe for the judge. (A black graduation robe or choir robe will work; companies that sell trophies and awards often have gavel sets.)

2. Prepare name tags for the other characters: defense attorney, prosecuting attorney, mother, father, IBCLC/RN, breast-feeding specialist, nursery nurse, pediatrician, office nurse, LLL leader, hospital administrator (CEO), insurance executive, and maternity unit manager. Optional characters: expert witness(es), formula company representative, state board of health official, and obstetrician.

---

[7] **Source:** This game was developed for the Lactation Consultant Exam Preparation Course formerly taught through Lact-Ed, Inc. ***This is a fictitious case. However, it is substantially based on real situations.***

Just before the session:

3. Select one student as the judge and two to fill the roles of the assistant prosecutor and assistant defense attorney. If two faculty members are available, one should assist the prosecutor and the other will assist the defense attorney. If only one instructor is available, she should coach both student-attorneys.

4. Arrange the room with a table and chair in the front for the judge, a witness chair, a table and chairs for the defense team and prosecution teams, a jury box with 12 chairs, a chair and table for the court reporter and/or bailiff, and chairs in the rear of the room for witnesses and observers (see diagram). Optional: Post *"Court Is In Session"* signs on the doors.

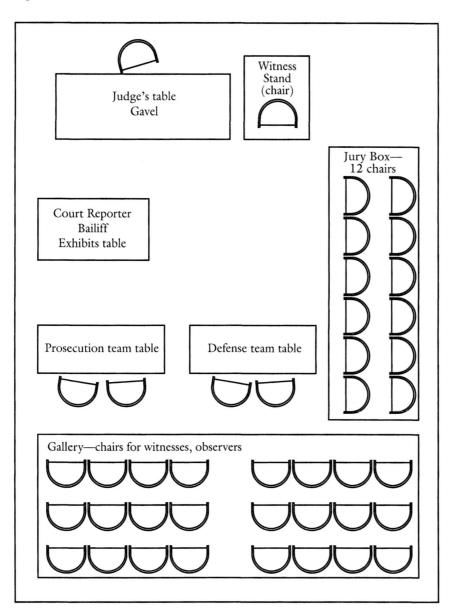

5. Place a witness name tag face down on as many of the seats as possible.

6. Provide a copy of the entire script and a description of the main characters for each student, and ask that they read it prior to this session. Provide a copy of the case sheets for the attorneys, bailiff, and judge at the start of the session.

7. Set out textbooks, monographs, and other documents that could be used as "evidence."

To begin the trial:

8. As the class convenes, have the judge put on the robe and wait outside the room until everyone else has arrived and has been seated. Arriving students, who were not preassigned a role, should be directed to the seats with name tags until all roles are filled. The mother, father, hospital administrator, and defense and prosecuting attorneys should move to their respective tables. The rest of the students should fill all the chairs in the jury box before filling the gallery. *The instructor must insist and assure that proper courtroom decorum is kept at all times.*

9. As soon as all students are in the room, the bailiff makes the announcement to open the trial. (See "order of events.")

10. Instructors should coach the student attorneys as needed. Try to address as many legal issues as possible during the emerging drama.

    Note: This game evolves a little differently almost every time it is played. There is plenty of blame to go around! The goal is to present a realistic drama, staying as close to the facts in the script as possible.

11. Instructor(s) should watch the time and allow at least 10–15 minutes for wrap-up and discussion after the trial ends. Instructors should address any other pertinent legal issues not brought up during the trial and discuss what went wrong.

    Teaching Tip: This game can have a profoundly unsettling, even shocking, effect on some students. The instructors should make themselves available for outside-of-class discussions and 1:1 counseling afterward. I usually schedule this game for an evening session midway through a several-day professional course.

MOCK TRIAL

Wrongful death of baby due to hypernatremic dehydration: The parents have filed a wrongful death suit against the hospital, the pediatrician, all nurses, and the lactation consultant (LC) involved and ask that the state investigate the hospital's lactation program. The hospital administrator (CEO) is the primary defendant.

Pertinent Information

The hospital has advertised a lactation program with classes, bedside rounds, and follow-up care.

The first-time mother has an epidural at 3 cm. after 12 hours of induction for postdates, pushes three hours, and delivers with help of a vacuum extractor. The baby weighs 8 lbs, 3 oz at birth; has APGAR scores of 6 and 9, and is deep suctioned in a radiant warmer; then goes to the nursery for observation for six hours. The baby first breastfeeds at six hours but doesn't latch. The LC sees the mother at eight hours to assist with positioning and latching; the baby feeds five minutes per side, and the LC instructs mother on frequency and duration of feeds, the prevention of sore nipples, and engorgement care. The baby's chart indicates that the baby "fed well" several times before discharge. A pacifier is placed in the baby's crib.

Mother and baby are discharged on a Friday, 28 hours post birth, with an ineffective manual breast pump provided by the hospital. Mother says the baby is not feeding well at discharge and was told not to worry because babies don't always feed well for the first few days; she was not instructed on pumping, feeding, stooling, or voiding. There is no planned follow-up by the hospital. A routine pediatric visit is scheduled for two weeks.

Day 4: Mother calls the maternity unit and talks to a "breastfeeding specialist." Mother is so engorged that the baby can't latch-on. The specialist instructs her to keep trying, use warm compresses, and reassures her that the baby eventually will go to breast, not to worry, and to avoid bottles. No documentation of this call exists.

Day 5: Mother calls the LLL Leader, who tells her to get in bed with the baby, get rid of visitors, hand-express to soften her breast before nursing, and to call the baby's doctor. The baby has not stooled since Day 3 and has had one wet diaper in the last 24 hours.

Day 6: Mother calls the hospital nursery again and says the baby's skin is dry, the baby is not feeding well, and the baby is hard to wake up. The hospital's LC refers the mother to her baby's pediatrician. The pediatrician's office nurse reassures the mother that some babies take a while to latch-on, that she should continue to try to breastfeed, and to keep the two-week appointment.

Day 7: Family members comment on the "good baby" who sleeps so much. The mother tries to awaken baby, who sucks three minutes per side and falls asleep every 4–5 hours. She calls the hospital to request a home visit and is told that her insurance plan does not include home visits for babies who fed well at discharge.

Day 8: The mother is desperate and is tempted to use the formula she received in her discharge pack, but is frightened because the baby "may be irrevocably harmed" and this will end her breastfeeding relationship. The mother goes back to the hospital, sees a nursery nurse, who gives her a nipple shield. The baby is still using a pacifier. Mother is instructed to waken baby every three hours for feeds.

Day 9: The baby has a seizure. Mother calls the pediatrician, who tells her to come in immediately. The pediatrician instructs the mother to "give formula" and sends her home. The mother is distraught; the father gives his baby 2 oz of undiluted concentrated formula every three hours.

Morning Day 11: The baby is found blue and cold in the crib. The parents file a wrongful death suit against the hospital, the pediatrician, all nurses, and the LC involved and ask the state to investigate the hospital's lactation program for fraud.

Witnesses for Mock Trial

IBCLC/RN works 15 hours as a LC and 25 hours as a staff nurse. She was certified three years ago and knows her stuff about lactation; she wishes she could devote full time to breastfeeding.

Breastfeeding specialist is a staff nurse who took a one-day course in breastfeeding and was "doing breastfeeding work" many years before the hospital hired the IBCLC/RN. She is jealous of IBCLC/RN, calls herself a specialist, and does not participate in continuing education programs in lactation because the hospital will not pay her way.

Pediatrician's spouse breastfed one child for three months with difficulty. He believes breast is best. He attended a continuing education program on infant feeding sponsored by a formula company three years ago.

Office nurse, no current experience with breastfeeding management but nursed two babies 25 years ago.

LLL Leader has one year of experience; her own baby is 2½ years old and still breastfeeds; she has no experience with early postpartum babies except her own and does not have a health-care background.

Mother is 26 years old, worked as secretary, completed two years of community college courses.

Father is 29 years old, works night shift at an automotive plant, and sleeps during the day. He is neither outwardly supportive nor unsupportive of breastfeeding.

Hospital administrator advertises Lactation Program for the public relations value. He resists the Baby Friendly Hospital Initiative™ (BFHI) program because the required staff training and purchasing of formula would be too costly to implement; he is worried that rooming-in will increase liability and is suspicious of mother support groups. (The hospital is Level II with a census of 2500 births annually.)

Insurance company or HMO executive is not convinced of the health benefits of breastfeeding and is reluctant to add home-care services for perinatal issues.

Other: Expert witness(es); formula company representative(s); State Board of Medicine/Health representative(s); LC's malpractice insurance agency underwriter

Order of Events for Mock Trial

1. Bailiff's announcement: "All rise, Court is now in session. Judge _____ is presiding." (Judge enters and is seated.) "You may be seated."

2. Opening statements
    a. Prosecutor: Provide summary of what you are going to present and prove.
    b. Defense: Provide summary of what you are going to present.

3. Prosecution witnesses
    a. Swearing-in: Witness places left hand on "bible" and right hand is raised. "Do you swear or affirm to tell the truth, the whole truth, and nothing but the truth? (Response). State your name for the court."
    b. Testimony is provided by witnesses.
    c. Cross-examination is conducted by defense.
    d. Objections
        1. Sustained = OK, which implies the objection was valid.
        2. Overruled = not OK, which implies the objection was not valid.

4. *Mid-trial recess: 10-minute break halfway through allotted time.* Judge will call attorneys to the bench for a "sidebar" conference and release all participants. Witnesses remain under oath; the jury is reminded to keep the proceedings confidential.

5. Defense witnesses are presented.
    a. Testimony is given.
    b. Cross-examination is conducted by prosecutor.

6. Closing statements are given by the following:
    a. Prosecutor
    b. Defense

7. The Judge gives instructions to the jury:
    a. Consider all facts presented here today.
    b. Disregard personal opinions or beliefs.
    c. Make a fair judgment based on the evidence.
    d. You may elect to make recommendations as well.

8. Jury deliberates and reaches a verdict, which they give to the Foreperson.

9. The verdict(s) are read and any recommendations from the Jury are heard.

10. Court is adjourned.

Class discussion begins. Refer to the legal issues list that follows and elaborate or expand as needed.

Legal Issues To Address during Mock Trial

- First do no harm

- Informed consent for all interventions including how baby and breastfeeding might be affected
  - Birth medications and procedures
  - Separation of mother and baby
  - Risk of discontinuation of breastfeeding/weaning to baby and mother

- Fraud; advertising something that is untrue

- Battery; unpermitted, intentional offense or harmful bodily contact

- Invasion of privacy

- Negligence

- Abandonment; care was discontinued without informing client

- Medical malpractice
  - Failure to diagnose
  - Failure to initiate treatment
  - Failure to refer or consult
  - Failure to provide attention or care
  - Failure to obtain informed consent
  - Provision of incorrect information resulting in illness/harm

- Nursing malpractice

- Failure to document

- Lactation Consultant malpractice

- Product liability

- Competency assurance and public protection

- Policies supportive of breastfeeding/ Baby Friendly Hospital Initiative ™

Prosecutor's Case

* Fraud— Hospital advertised services that did not exist, exaggerated, and increased rates to cover expanded services.

* Negligence—Hospital failed to ensure follow-up care within 48 hours of discharge according to Joint Perinatal Guidelines. (Argument is weak because the physician discharges the baby, but the hospital extends privileges to the physician.)

* Malpractice—Nurses failed to document, especially telephone calls.

* Malpractice—Pediatrician failed to diagnose dehydration and appropriately treat. Inadequate follow-up care was provided; the pediatrician failed to follow AAP guidelines on early follow-up for breastfed babies.

* Malpractice—Failed to obtain informed consent for childbirth medications, feeding devices, and formula.

* Battery—Nurse put a bottle of glucose water in the baby's bassinette when parents specifically said "no supplements."

* Product liability—Nurse did not use a product (tube feeder) according to the manufacturer's written instructions, which did not cover using the product at breast. Product liability laws also apply to use of peridontal syringes, nasogastric tubes, nipple pullers, etc.

* Ethical issues——The Hospital advertised services that were not supported by appropriate job descriptions, sufficient pay, and appropriate requirements for staff; "gifts" were accepted from formula companies, and insufficient staff training was provided.

Defense Attorney's Case

* Blame someone else, especially the pediatrician. (Argument is weak, because the pediatrician still has hospital privileges.)

* We've had consistently good evaluations from State Maternity Licensing Unit and/or JCAHO (Argument is weak, because neither organization thoroughly addresses breast-feeding management.)

* Tragic errors were made by mother, dad, nurses, and doctor, but all actions are within published standards.

* We were not required to have any of these services; we've gone "above and beyond" the minimum requirements.

* Our responsibility ended when the baby was discharged.

* We made good faith efforts to help.

* Parents signed consent at admission; mothers often are over-anxious; the hospital staff gave sufficient information during the stay and at discharge.

* Baby Friendly Hospital Initiative™ is voluntary, costly, and we've been warned not to implement it because of restraint-of-trade issues.

What Went Wrong?

* Incorrect information

* No informed consent

* No policy/standards of care

* Inappropriate follow-up

* Inadequate staff

* Inadequate training

* False advertising

* Failure to refer/collaborate

* Inadequate/confusing labels

* Falsifying records (?)

* Inadequate/poor documentation

* No continuity of care

* Lack of professional integrity

* Poor communication

MYSTERY GAME [8]

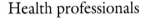

GOAL

To learn methods of identifying and solving common breastfeeding problems

BEST AUDIENCE
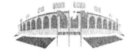

Health professionals

TIME REQUIRED

20–30 minutes for four mysteries

HOW TO PLAY

Make two identical sets of clue cards: four cards per case, and four mystery cases. (One case for about six people; four cases is about right for 50 people.) Each of the four clues per case gives a piece of information relevant to the mother, baby, or both. Some cases should be easy to assess; others should be more vague or complicated; and some may not even indicate a problem.

Divide the class into groups; each group gets a set of cards, which are shuffled and dealt. Whoever holds a clue card for that case reads it until all four clues are read. Then the group discusses the problem and proposes interventions if appropriate. One person in each group acts as recorder. Groups with the same case take turns reporting what they found and what they would do about it. A listening group with the same case gets to critique the other group's findings. The instructor comments, expands, and corrects information presented.

[8] **Source:** This game is adapted from "The Labor Mystery," which I first learned from Suzanne Hilbers, RPT, FACCE.

SUGGESTED CASES

* Kathryn is having bright red lochial discharge; her baby, Paul, wants to nurse 10–15 times a day and seems to be hungry after nursings; Paul was born to Kathryn weighing 8 lbs, 1 oz. Today, he weighs 7 lbs, 14 oz; Paul is 2½ weeks old. (*Problem:* Retained placenta resulting in suppressed lactation. *Solution:* She needs a dilation and curettage procedure [D&C.])

* Tomika's mother, Cherese, complains that her right breast is red, hot, and swollen; Cherese's nipples are very sore in the center of the nipple tip; Tomika's tongue is heart-shaped at the tip; Tomika, Cherese's baby, is four days old. She was born by cesarean section with epidural anesthesia. (*Problem:* Baby is tongue-tied baby [ankyloglossia] and can't remove milk effectively; mother is developing mastitis. *Solution:* Arrange for the baby's frenulum to be clipped (frenotomy); help the mother get started with pumping and cup-feeding her baby.)

* Charlene went back to work at her job as a chemist at an oil refinery last week; Charlene suddenly developed sore, itchy nipples; Charlene's baby Todd is two months old; Charlene collects milk for Todd with an inexpensive battery-operated pump. (*Problem:* Nipple thrush (candida). *Solution:* Assure that the mother and baby are treated for thrush simultaneously; also check on the volume of milk collected with this pump.)

* Jenny's baby, Amber, is 12 days old and weighs 6 lbs 2 oz; Amber wets 8–10 diapers and has 3–4 loose yellow stools every day; Amber nurses about every hour for 10–15 minutes; Amber only nurses on one of Jenny's breasts per feeding. (*Problem:* None; this is normal behavior. *Solution:* Reassure the mother and refer her to a mother support group.)

THE SNAKE OIL SHOW[9]

GOAL

To learn principles of pharmacokinesis—how drugs taken by a lactating mother transfer into her milk

BEST AUDIENCE
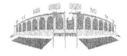

Health care professionals and LC students

TIME REQUIRED

About 90 minutes

HOW TO PLAY

Make up at least one set of Category/Principle cards. A set of 16 cards should contain the following:

- Four *Absorption Category* principle cards, all the same color:
  - Protein binding
  - Lipid solubility
  - Molecular weight
  - Active metabolites
- Four *Distribution Category* principle cards, all the same color, but a different color from the other categories
  - Milk:plasma ratio
  - pH (acid/base rating)
  - Ionization
  - Destruction in the gut

---

[9] **Source:** This game was developed for the *Lactation Consultant Exam Preparation Course* formerly taught through Lact-Ed, Inc.

124

* Three *Elimination Category* principle cards, all the same color, but a different color from the other categories

    – Metabolism

    – Half-life (T ½)

    – Time to peak level

* Five *Compatibility Category* principle cards, all the same color, but a different color from the other categories:

    – Age of baby

    – A.A.P. categories

    – Pediatric dose

    – Risks of weaning

    – Alternatives; delay

Make sure that pharmacology reference materials are available in the classroom, such as *Breastfeeding, a Guide for the Medical Profession* by Lawrence & Lawrence, and *Medications and Mothers' Milk* by Thomas Hale.

Distribute the cards so that each person gets one principle to research (one card) and every principle is researched by at least one person. If more than 16 people are playing, have more than one person research each principle. If fewer than 16 are playing, assign two people to work on three principles so that nobody has to work on two principles alone. Students can research these principles on their own or team up with others with the same color (Category) cards.

Instructions can be printed on the reverse side of each card.

* *Part 1:* The color of this card represents one *category* of drug actions and lists one *principle* of whether and how drugs taken by a lactating mother may affect her nursing baby. Take a few minutes to look up this *one principle only*, even though you may learn about other related principles in the process.

* *Part 2:* Get together with others in the same Category (those who have similar color cards). Each Category has three to five principles. Your Category group will now devise a simple, brief presentation to illustrate the Category and all its principles to a grade-school audience. Do not focus on specific drugs, except as examples.

* Feel free to be creative. Presentations can be skits, games, songs, drawings, show-and-tell with household or kitchen items, etc. The presentation should be brief—no more than a few minutes long. Use any props, teaching materials, or other items that you can find to illustrate your Category and the principles.

Announce the time that presentations will begin. Explain that you will make sure that all the pertinent information gets covered (and covered accurately) in some manner. If incorrect information is given, gently make the correction without embarrassing the presenters (if possible). After all groups have given their presentations, address any questions that arose during this exercise. Supplement with handouts, discussion, and overheads as needed.

Teaching Tips

* Allow about 20–30 minutes for Part 1. Circulate and assist as needed. This part is "open book," so help students find this information. Don't explain the principle completely; knowing where to find the information is one goal of the exercise. Students inevitably learn more than their assigned principle.

* Allow about 20–30 minutes for Part 2. Again, circulate and assist as needed. Offer any classroom equipment/supplies that the groups might want to use.

* Some groups try to turn this into a college-level lecture. Remind them that the intended audience is sixth grade children; this will keep the game simpler and more fun.

Bonus #1:

One class team developed a Jeopardy™-like game to explain *Half-life* and *Metabolism*. Here are their game questions:

1. Category (Principle) Half-Life

   - For 100 points, true or false: The longer the half-life of the drug, the greater the risk of accumulation in the mother or infant. **True**

   - For 200 points, true or false: All drugs have very similar half-lives. **False**

   - For 300 points, answer A, B, or C: Half-life is (A) the time it takes for a drug to double in strength; (B) the break between two halves of a football game; or (C) the time it takes the serum concentration to decrease by one half. **C**

   - For 400 points, answer A, B, or C: Half-life is determined by (A) the amount of milk a mother pumps from her breast and then discards; (B) the amount of antibiotics passed through maternal milk; or (C) the drug's rates of absorption, metabolism, and excretion from the body. **C**

   - For 500 points, answer A, B, or C: A drug with a short half-life is taken (A) more frequently; (B) less frequently; or (C) whenever wanted. **A**

2. Category (Principle) Metabolism

   - For 100 points, answer A, B, or C: Drugs are generally detoxified and conjugated by which organ? (A) brain; (B) liver; or (C) mouth. **B**

- For 200 points, true or false: A drug considered compatible for a term breastfeeding baby will also be safe for a preemie. **False;** not always

- For 300 points, true or false: Renal clearance is not affected by the maturity of the infant. **False**

- For 400 points, answer A, B, or C: At about _____ weeks conceptual age, an infant's liver is able to metabolize most drugs competently. (A) 38 weeks; (B) 40 weeks; (C) 42 weeks. **C**

- For 500 points, true or false: Most compounds that appear in milk in very low levels are easily excreted by the infant. **False**

Bonus #2:

YOUNG MS. DONALD TOOK A DRUG

(Distribution Category)[10]

(Sung to the tune of "Old McDonald Had a Farm")

Young Ms. Donald took a drug, E-I-E-I-O
And for that drug to be safe
She needs to know some things.

Was it an acid? Was it a base? A charged-up acid slows the pace
Young Ms. Donald took a drug, E-I-E-I-O!

Bind it up here, bind it up there,
Ship it to the gut, Chomp Chomp Chomp!
Young Ms. Donald had some milk, E-I-E-I-O!
Less in the blood, a little in the milk,
Sucking at the breast; that's the best!
Young Ms. Donald had awesome milk, E-I-E-I O!

Bonus #3:

Pharmacology principles can be made into crossword puzzles or word search games. Software programs will help with preparation.

---

[10] **Source:** This song/skit was written and choreographed by Deborah Swiger, Sherry Sommers, Kathi Jones, Marie Cobb, Gail Sevy, and Kim Gorsuch (with her baby Hailey) on April 25, 1999, in Cincinnati, Ohio.

SLEEPING THROUGH

GOAL

To explore infant sleep needs and patterns in the context of adult experiences

BEST AUDIENCE

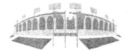

Groups of at least 10 people—parents or professionals

TIME REQUIRED

10–20 minutes

HOW TO PLAY

Everyone needs paper and pencil. Have students write down the answers to the following:

1. How long do you sleep at night, in total?

2. How many times do you wake up during that time?

3. What do you do when you wake at night? (Go to the rest room, eat something, drink water, and so on)

4. Does anyone or anything share your bed—spouse, pet, or other object?

5. What conditions allow you to sleep best?

6. What conditions make it most difficult for you to sleep?

Analyze the answers and correlate them to infant sleep. The pertinent points are

- Few people can sleep when they're not sleepy.

- Fear, loneliness, and hunger will interfere with sleep.

* Strange smells or sounds interfere with sleep.

* Many adults sleep better with their spouse or partner. Babies sleep better with their mothers in physical contact with them.

Sleep training philosophies and programs interfere with appropriate nighttime breastfeeding behaviors. I took the elements of sleep training strategies and developed this "Sleep Training for Newlyweds" program. The point is to illustrate how ridiculous these strategies are for a newly married couple. Because babies need the physical touch of their mothers, including at night, my goal is to show the inappropriateness of these strategies for babies.

- Make sure that your new spouse sleeps in a separate bedroom. You wouldn't want him to get too dependent on you.

- Put him to sleep alone, on a schedule.

- Develop a bedtime routine, with rituals that will help him prepare for sleep.

- Get him a comfort object, such as a teddy bear or other stuffed toy.

- Take him on a car ride before bed to help him relax. He may even fall asleep in the car, and you can take him to his room without disturbing his sleep.

- Play soothing music, sing him to sleep, or play tapes of waterfalls or gentle surf sounds.

- Leave a night-light on for reassurance.

- Get him soft blankets to make his bed a cozy, comfortable place.

- If he protests that he's lonely without you, don't give in. Let him cry it out a few nights so that he learns not to manipulate you.

- If you have to go in to his room at night, limit touching because it rewards his crying out for you and encourages more wakefulness.

- If he tries to come into your room at night, block or lock the door.

- Make sure that he eats right before bed so that he doesn't wake because of hunger, but don't let him drink large quantities of liquid, or he'll wake to void.

- Give him plenty of attention, affection, and stimulation during the daytime to lessen his desire to be with you at night.

Teaching Tip: This game does not work every time or for all audiences. Some people are uncomfortable with the idea that the baby's need for physical contact with mother is being compared to the marital relationship. If this objection surfaces, focus on the need/desire for physical touch, not adult sexual behaviors.

SUCKLE UP[11]

· ·

GOAL

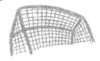

To teach infant suck by simulating physical/mechanical aspects of infant suck and milk transfer using household items

BEST AUDIENCE

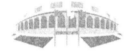

Health care professionals and lactation management students

TIME REQUIRED

90 minutes

HOW TO PLAY

Equipment needed:

* Bland flavored crackers, such as saltines, two crackers per student. Be aware of any dietary restrictions (wheat allergies, Kosher) of the group members.

* Straws, preferably individually wrapped, one each

* Small cups or drinking glasses (eight oz or less), one each

* Small disposable squirt guns, such as those sold as party favors, one each

* Three to four squirt guns of different sizes (and force of water stream)

* Small household funnels in several sizes, at least three for the entire group.

* Pitchers of water

---

[11] **Source:** This game was developed for the *Lactation Consultant Exam Preparation Course* formerly taught through Lact-Ed, Inc.

Part 1:

1. Chew and swallow one of the crackers without drinking any water to wash it down. Pay attention to the changing texture of the cracker, how your tongue moves the material around in your mouth, your breathing, and what your jaws do.

2. Pour some water into your cup. Using one of the straws, take a few sips of water through the straw. Pay attention to where the straw tip rests in your mouth, what your tongue and lips do, and your breathing. Experiment with straw placement in your mouth to see what happens with your tongue, lips, and jaws.

3. Using the open cup, drink a little water. Again, pay attention to the placement of the cup against your lips, what your tongue and jaws are doing, the angle of your head, and your breathing.

4. *Discussion:* Analyze the differences in these different foods/fluids, tongue motion, and breathing and compare these to infant feeding. The crackers are somewhat like colostrum, a thick almost gel-like substance. Be sure to compare breathing patterns with swallowing.

Part 2:

Fill your squirt guns with water. Team up with a partner and swap so that your partner will be squirting you with your own gun.

1. First, open your mouth wide while your partner squirts water (from your own squirt gun) into your mouth from an arm's length away (about 2 feet). Observe what your tongue, lips, and jaws do with the water and how you manage to swallow and breathe. Then repeat the exercise with your partner being the recipient.

2. Second, put the tip of your squirt gun in your mouth, and purse your lips tightly around the barrel. Squirt it a few times. Observe what your tongue, lips, and jaws do with the water and how you manage to swallow and breathe.

3. Third, again put the squirt gun in your mouth, but this time place your lips loosely around the barrel. Repeat the exercise, again observing what your tongue, lips, and jaws do with the water and how you manage to swallow and breathe.

4. *Discussion:* Analyze the differences in the flow rate and what affect your mouth and lips have on the ability to capture (control) the liquid, swallow, and breathe. Most people find that relaxed lips result in the best control of the liquid. The squirt guns illustrate milk letting-down and the baby positioned in various ways at the breast.

Bonus: Fill the additional squirt guns and then squirt some water with each. This illustrates that the milk will flow or spray with differing intensity or force. Milk flow velocity will affect how the baby will handle milk flow. Discuss the physiology of let-down and milk ejection reflex.

Part 3:

Ask for two volunteers for each funnel.

1. The recipient should lean back in a chair so that her head is neither flexed nor extended and her mouth is pointed toward the ceiling. She places a funnel in her mouth, using her hands to adjust the placement of the tip inside her mouth.

2. Using a pitcher or cup, the server slowly pours water into the funnel. Continue until one to two ounces have been poured. Watch the recipient carefully, matching the flow of water to the recipient's comfort and ability to swallow the incoming water.

3. *Discussion:* Both recipient and server describe what it was like for them, including the emotional aspects. The recipient describes what she did with her tongue and the funnel placement to control the flow and to allow breathing. The server describes what she watched for. Correlate this to using a feeding bottle and teat to provide milk to the baby and what the baby must do to compensate.

YOUR TEENAGERS GAME

GOAL

To really understand the importance of mother and baby being together early and often to achieve a mutually loving and trusting interaction

BEST AUDIENCE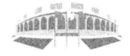

Adults (parents and professionals)

TIME REQUIRED

30 minutes (10 minutes for each phase)

HOW TO PLAY

Divide the group into teams of three to six players; the different genders should be separate if possible. This game also can be played as one large group.

Equipment needed: Each team needs paper and pencil. Or, the instructor or facilitator can record answers on an overhead, newsprint pad, etc.

Phase one: Imagine that your hot-blooded, romantic 16-year-old son or daughter is dating a very unsavory person. List all the ways you can discourage their romance and keep them from becoming intimate. When finished, the groups report back on strategies they have invented, which usually will include physical separation, forced new friends, lack of privacy, disparaging remarks, scare tactics, and so on. Cut the list down to the top five and then the top two and then the number-one bottom-line strategy to prevent them from becoming physically intimate.

Phase two: Remember when *you* were falling in love with your partner, leading up to your honeymoon. List all the ways you can imagine

133

that someone could help (or did help) you fall in love and become physically intimate. When finished, groups report back. These reports will usually include privacy, complimentary remarks, body contact, sufficient time together, etc. Cut the list down to the top five, and then two, and then the number-one strategy for physical intimacy.

Phase three: Discuss both aspects as they relate to the need for a mother and baby to become physically intimate in order for breastfeeding to work, starting immediately at birth.

When finished, commit to at least one concrete thing you can do *in the next two weeks* to help mothers and babies become more intimate. Write this down on something you can take home. If you are a parent, you can implement this idea immediately. If you are a staff member, pick something you have the authority and ability to do immediately. Staff members should also include strategies to make this commitment a permanent part of unit routines for all staff members.

5
SECRETS
OF THE PROS

Neat and Nifty Ideas
from Master Teachers

BALLOON SANDWICHES[1]

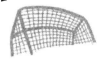

GOAL

To simulate latch techniques using balloons

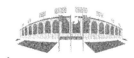

BEST AUDIENCE

All, especially health care professionals and lactation-management students

TIME REQUIRED

10–20 minutes

Warning: This exercise uses latex balloons and involves students putting the balloons into their mouths. Announce these aspects beforehand and make it easy for any student to avoid participation for medical or personal reasons. Use only new helium-quality balloons, which are resistant to breakage. Warn participants not to bite down, and that participation is at their own risk.

HOW TO PLAY

One balloon is needed for each participant. Use helium-quality 6–9-inch diameter balloons in light colors, such as white, yellow, or pink. Avoid dark colors.

Bright shades or dark red lipsticks are also needed; avoid pale shades. Students may use their own lipsticks. Have available several extra tubes plus cotton swabs for applying.

Have students blow up their balloons to the size of a breast. This instruction usually draws questions about what's normal, which is a great opportunity to discuss mammary anatomy! Tie the ends securely.

---

[1] **Source:** Diane Wiessinger, MA, IBCLC. This description is adapted from Wiessinger, D. A breastfeeding teaching tool using a sandwich analogy for latch-on. *J Hum Lact* 1998; 14(1): 51–56. Please refer to the article for more details, the game's application to clinical practice, and pictures of Diane's technique.

* If tap water is easily available, invite students to partly fill their balloons with warm water.

* Remind the group that these balloons are *not* for throwing at each other!

First try: Centered latch. Apply some lipstick to your lips and open wide. Now aim the end of the balloon (the part farthest away from the knot) directly at the center of your mouth. Bring it to your mouth, placing your lips firmly on the surface. (*Optional:* Suck gently on the balloon, allowing it to stretch into your mouth a little. **Do not bite down**.) Remove your lips from the balloon and note the location of your lipstick marks.

Second try: Sandwich latch. Apply more lipstick. This time, holding the balloon in two hands as you would a large sandwich, compress (flatten) the balloon in a straight line parallel to your upper lip. Repeat the latch onto the flattened balloon. Note that the lipstick marks from this attempt indicate that *more* of the balloon got into your mouth.

Third try: Sandwich technique plus off-centered latch. Apply more lipstick and compress (flatten) the balloon again. Start with the balloon below the level of your chin, with the end pointing at your nose. Open wide and bring the balloon sandwich up and over your lower lip, rotating the end of the balloon toward the center of your mouth as you bring it upward and toward your mouth. Use your lower lip as a pivot. Repeat the latch. Note from the lipstick marks that *even more* of the balloon was inside your mouth.

Discuss the differences in these techniques and their implications to mothers. If anyone sucked gently on the balloon, have that person describe the differences.

BELLY STONES[2]

GOAL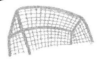

To understand infant feeding by simulating stomach capacity of the infant

BEST AUDIENCE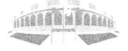

All

TIME REQUIRED

A few minutes

HOW TO PLAY

Collect various sizes of polished stones (rocks or minerals), household objects, food items, and so on to represent the capacity of the stomach at different ages.

Age	Size of Stomach	Comparable Objects
1 day	5–7 ml	Hazelnut, cooked chick pea, thimble, glass marble
3 days	22–27 (about 1 oz)	Ordinary teaspoon, malted milk ball, drawing of baby's fist
10 days	45–60 ml (1½–2 oz)	Walnut, golf ball, coffee measuring scoop
Adult	900 ml (2 cups)	Softball, grapefruit, measuring cup, drawing of adult fist

When discussing how often babies need to eat, pass around the objects to illustrate the baby's need for frequent feeds.

Another approach is to display a marble, golf ball, and tennis ball or softball. Have students guess which represents the baby's stomach capacity at birth (marble) and at about 10 days (golf ball). The tennis ball or softball is the size of an adult stomach.

[2] References:

Scammon RE and Doyle LO. Observations on the capacity of the stomach in the first ten days of postnatal life. *Am J Dis. Child*, 1920; 20: 516–538.

Silverman, MA, ed. *Dunman's Premature Infants*, 3rd edition. New York: Hoeber, Inc., Medical Division of Harper and Brothers, 1961, p. 143–144.

BRILLIANT PLAYS: ANALOGIES AND METAPHORS

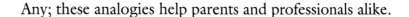

GOAL

Compare aspects of breastfeeding to other life events and activities

BEST AUDIENCE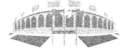

Any; these analogies help parents and professionals alike.

TIME REQUIRED

Varies

HOW TO PLAY

Work these analogies into breastfeeding classes, courses, and discussions.

* Breastfeeding is like learning to dance. At first, the partners move awkwardly, sometimes stepping on one another's toes and fighting for the lead. With time and practice, they learn to read and anticipate each other's movements and strengths. Their movements smooth out and become fluid as they become more skilled. Each partner becomes more confident in his or her ability to interact positively and comfortably with the other.

    —Many sources

* This analogy is for women who want to do both breastfeeding and bottle-feeding from birth. Doing both is like having a roller skate on one foot and an ice skate on the other. You won't get very far. It's better to learn one way and make it easy (for mother and baby) before learning another way.

    —Nikki Lee RN, MSN, mother of two, IBCLC, CIMI, CSTP; Elkins Park, PA

* When moms ask, "Gosh, will it take a LOOOOOOONG time to fix this problem?" and the baby is 10 days old, offer up this analogy: Suppose that you break your leg. You go to the hospital, and they propose to cast it. The doctor says it will take six weeks to heal enough to take the cast off, and then it will take more time to completely heal after that. Do you look at the doctor and say, "Heck no, I can't wait that long, just cut it off?" When you have a breastfeeding problem, it may take time to fix the problem, but it's worth it.

—Carol Brussel, IBCLC; Denver, CO

* Learning to drive a car is easier with someone sitting beside you to help. When you were first married, you had to work together until things went smoothly. When you learned to ride a bike, you fell many times until you got the hang of it and could do it without thinking.

—Laurie Wheeler, RN, MN, IBCLC; Violet, LA

* For moms who have partial milk supplies and want to switch to total formula: If you ate junk food for some meals, it would still be worth it to have home-cooked, nutritionally sound meals for even one meal a day. You would not say, "Oh well, I'll just go totally over to junk food."

—Laurie Wheeler, RN, MN, IBCLC; Violet, LA

* I often use the words "bunch of grapes" when I explain milk synthesis to a mother. The alveoli are the "bunch," and one milk-producing cell is a single grape. (Sometimes these cells are referred to as a "single milk factory," but I don't like to use the word "factory" in this context.) Imagine what happens when those myoepithelial cells contract (i.e., squeeze the grape). Here's your milk ejection reflex!

—Renate J. M. Rietveld, IBCLC; Rijswijk, The Netherlands

* My husband is a great advocate of breastfeeding and will tell all his relatives and friends, who are unaware of the benefits of breastfeeding, "Breastmilk is like beer (something many men enjoy). Would you rather drink it 'on tap' or from a can?" Many men smile and nod when he says this.

—Heidi Roibal, BS, LLLL; Albuquerque, NM

* To help a mom understand why her baby takes so long to feed or gets frustrated and gives up, when latch is poor, I tell her what Freda Rosenfeld shared with me: It's like riding a bicycle when the chain keeps slipping; you might keep having to start over; you work harder than you would if the chain was on right; you are more likely to get frustrated; you might get where you are going, but it takes a lot longer than usual; and you might be more likely to need more breaks on the way there.

—Judy LeVan Fram; Brooklyn, NY

* I use the same analogy mentioned by another Lactnetter to explain the need for hindmilk, but I take it one step further. I tell parents that getting only foremilk is like sitting down at every meal and drinking a glass of juice and leaving the food on your plate. You will become hungry very soon after the meal, and worse yet, the cook will no longer bother to prepare a full meal for you.

—Jennifer Tow, IBCLC; Glastonbury, CT

* Learning to breastfeed is like learning to ride a two-wheel bike. It can be difficult and takes practice. Bottle-feeding is more like learning to ride a tricycle. A tricycle is easy to learn, usually you can the first time you try. After breastfeeding is learned, however, it is so much better than bottle-feeding, sort of like how much faster and farther you can go on a bicycle versus a tricycle.

—Tracy Throckmorton RN, IBCLC; Lake Oswego, OR

* After mom's milk volume really kicks in, after a couple of days the baby may be overwhelmed with the increased flow. I liken this to drinking from a drinking fountain when the water pressure increases (or someone plays a trick by turning it up). I find that almost everyone has had this happen to them at some point in their lives, and they can really relate to a baby's possible reaction.

—Winnie Mading, IBCLC; Sussex, WI

* Here is an example for engorgement: Imagine that your breast is a balloon. As your breast fills with milk, it is a lot like a balloon filling with air. The "nipple" on the end of the balloon will protrude nicely to demonstrate proper latch. The balloon initially looks like it has a nipple, but as it fills up, the nipple flattens. Milk pools behind the areolar tissue, and as a result, your nipple becomes flatter, and it becomes more difficult for the baby to latch. Expressing some milk for the baby to have a supple nipple to latch onto can facilitate the feed.

—Debbie Albert, PhD, IBCLC; Tampa, FL and Heidi S. Roibal; Albuquerque, NM

* When baby is not latched well, he doesn't get much; it's like sucking through a straw with a hole in the side of it—very frustrating and unsatisfying. However, when the straw is intact, you get a good mouthful of fluid, and it satisfies you.

—Laurie Wheeler, RN, MN, IBCLC; Violet, LA

* Some mothers with perceived milk insufficiency will tell me that they "wait until the breasts are full" before nursing. The metaphor I like to use in this case is that it's like saying that you're out of breath, but are going to "wait until your lungs are full of air" before breathing. (This analogy always gets me a laugh.) Then I make the point that just like the act of breathing is what brings oxygen into the lungs, it is the act of nursing that produces milk, not the other way around. I use lungs as metaphors for breasts quite a lot, and other organs generally. Sometimes I'll treat the subject with

a bit of humor: "Breasts are a lot like lungs," I'll say. "You've got two of them; you have to use them often, or they won't work; and there's no limit to how often they can be used!"

—Regina Roig Lane, BS IBCLC; Miami, FL

* Does anyone ever come up to a pregnant woman and say, "Your placenta isn't strong enough?" You trusted your body to make this beautiful baby from those two little cells so long ago—your body knew exactly what to do—why should it suddenly get it wrong now? Does anyone ever question you about frequent feeding in the early hours or days? Your baby was being "drip fed" continuously through the umbilical cord a few hours ago, and suddenly along we come and cut off his food supply and then expect him to go from continuous feeding to eating every few hours. He will take time to get used to an intermittent food supply. He has also lots of new things happening to him that probably frighten him, and you are his security; you are the only thing he is used to, so he needs to be really close to you so that you can protect him; he trusts you. And my personal favorite!: Has anyone ever said to you, "You've lost your milk." "Where do you think you might have left it? Shall I help you look for it? Is it under the bed, or did you leave it in the bathroom?" That one seems to really hit home as to how silly the concept is! I use this one when preparing mums for the "outside world!"

—Susan Kay, midwife; Australia

* I used to describe foremilk/hindmilk as a glass of lemonade and a sandwich. The glass of lemonade will satisfy your thirst and fill your belly for a while, but the sandwich will keep you satisfied for hours.

—Kirsten Blacker, RN, RM; Gwelup, Australia

* I tell moms that teaching children to nurse is like teaching them to drive; if you don't teach them right, you get hurt. And, just as you don't expect your child to learn to drive overnight, sometimes it takes weeks to learn to nurse!

—Christine M. Betzold, MSN, NP, CLE; Garden Grove, CA

* Here in Northern California many people have wood stoves and need a chainsaw. I compare buying breast pumps to buying chainsaws. People pay lots of money for a good chainsaw because they want it to be safe and efficient. I tell my classes that we are looking for the same qualities in a breast pump—safety and efficiency—and we may have to pay more for a good one. The men in the group can really relate.

—Star Siegfried RN, BA, IBCLC; Arcata, CA

* I use this metaphor when mothers can't seem to believe that breastfed babies are "supposed" to eat more often than bottle-fed babies. We have a real problem here with mothers thinking that the only definition of a well-fed baby is that he not eat more often than every 3–4 hours. For that kind of mom, I'll say something along these lines: Suppose that your neighbor (friend, whoever) and you had dinner together at a restaurant. You

had a steak, a baked potato with butter and sour cream, a vegetable, and a piece of key lime pie for dessert. (We are in Miami after all, where key lime pies *rule.*) Your friend had a pasta salad with lots of little crunchy raw veggies in the salad, a little skinless chicken breast, and perhaps some fruit for dessert. "Which one of you is going to be hungry first?" I ask. The answer that *always* comes back to me is Miss Pasta Salad. "Does that mean that your friend didn't eat enough? Does it mean that there was something wrong with her food? Does it mean that what she chose to eat was nutritionally inadequate?" No! It simply means that she had a lighter meal than you did, one that is likely to be digested more quickly than your steak, baked potato, sour cream, and pie. "Formula is the steak and baked potato," I tell them. "Breastmilk is the pasta salad. It's wonderful food, tasty, nutritious, and a lot healthier than that steak. You're better off eating the pasta salad. But, it's not going to sit in your stomach for as long as the steak will." That usually makes my point that it's *normal* for a breastfed baby to eat more often than an artificially fed one.

—Regina Roig Lane, BS, IBCLC; Miami, FL

* Learning to breastfeed can be like learning how to walk. Your child will try, and try, and try again to take that first step. He'll fall any number of times in the process. After he takes that first step, no one cares or remembers how many times he fell, only that he finally took that first step! Also, no one expects him never to fall again. Instead, what they expect is that each day he'll fall less than he did the day before. We expect persistence from our kids in learning how to walk. We need that same persistence and positive attitude in teaching them how to breastfeed.

—Regina Roig Lane, BS, IBCLC; Miami, FL

* I compare the breastfeeding and bottle-feeding to learning to drive a car with standard transmission (breastfeeding) and learning to drive a car with automatic transmission (bottle). I explain that after you learn to drive a standard, you are good to go on anything. I ask them how many people they know who learned on automatic want anything to do with driving a standard.

—Barb Berges BS, RN, IBCLC; Rochester, NY

* When talking about breast milk production, I refer to the alveoli and duct system as being like broccoli in shape. This helps students to visualize the clusters well. I use the standard breast structure diagram with this talk. I like to give them a clear visualization of the breast structure to explain the nature of engorgement and it's prevention and treatment. Breastfed babies are not gas tanks. They do not go from full to empty and then get a fill up. I explain that babies can be trained (forced, coerced) to get into this mode with bottles of formula that digest slowly. However, babies are meant to be more like us grownups. We eat when we are hungry, and drink when we are thirsty, and we don't watch the clock. I then go into the "buffet" style of eating to explain cluster feeding: we have a little salad, then have some main course, socialize with our friends, eat a few desserts, linger over coffee, and then not eat again for hours. Mums and dads seem

to identify well with this idea and see that their babies are more like themselves rather than strange, unroutined little aliens who never seem satisfied.

—Janet Vandenberg RN, BScN, IBCLC; Newmarket, ON

* One analogy that I use with prenatal breastfeeding classes I borrowed from a breast-feeding book, one of the authors may have been Renfrew. The cartoon in the book shows that BF is like learning to drive a car (most everyone in this area drives). I explain that when you first learn to drive, you concentrate on each step: adjust the seat, adjust the rear view mirror, put the car in gear, turn the key, step on the gas, step on the brake, change gears, etc. Now when you drive, you don't think about each step; it's automatic; it's easy to drive. When you first breastfeed, you concentrate on each step: position yourself, position baby, support breast, tickle baby's mouth, wait for open mouth, pull baby quickly onto breast, etc. After you and the baby have learned to do it, it's automatic; it's easy to breastfeed.

—Laura Hart, RN, BSN, IBCLC; Winter Park, FL

* When learning to breastfeed: Remember your first sexual experience. It was pretty much a disaster, but when you had more practice together, it got better. (Choose recipients carefully for this one!) Or, for more reserved clients: Remember when you learned to drive a car, you had to put your hands here, sit this way, and put your feet there. It took a while to learn, but now it comes automatically.

—Susan Kay, RN, RM, BN, IBCLC; Toowoomba, Australia

* I really enjoyed the lung metaphors, but then I began to think. . . . I never doubt my lungs or my stomach will work, but I also didn't doubt that my uterus would work and help me give birth to a baby in the usual way. However, it didn't, even with all the things folks tried to prod it along, so I had a cesarean. At the time I remember thinking angrily that my body had *failed* me, like I could never trust it again. So, is the lung metaphor not a good one to use on women who experienced cesarean births? No, I don't think so, because upon further thought, I said to myself, "Hmmm, if my breathing were put in an unfamiliar place, with people scrutinizing the efficiency and power of each breath, measuring them to be sure they are "good enough," giving medications to make the breaths stronger and more efficient, making me scared and nervous, etc., maybe my breathing *would* get confused and erratic. Just like my uterus had been. Breastfeeding, on the other hand, is a natural thing where *you* are in control, and even if there are problems, you are in the loving hands of your LC or lay practitioner. Seeing how well breastfeeding goes can help mothers who have experienced something other than their ideal version of childbirth to learn that they *do* have powerful, wonderful bodies. So, you have to stretch the metaphor a bit, but I think it still works. Personally, I sure am glad that I successfully breastfed; it really did make up for the birth experiences.

—Sue Ann Kendall, MA, LLLL; Austin, TX

* I used my favorite analogy just last week with a young couple. The mom asked me whether it was okay to hold her baby a lot, because her husband and his family keep telling her to let the baby cry or it will be spoiled. The husband seemed a little slow and didn't seem too impressed by my "studies have shown that you can't spoil a baby" explanation. So I tried, "Imagine you lived all of your life in Jamaica where it is warm everyday and people speak one language. Now imagine you woke up one day, and you were in the North Pole, and you didn't know where you were or how you got there, and you couldn't ask because no one understood you. Wouldn't you be a little scared? Now imagine that you recognized one person. . . . Wouldn't you kind of "cling" to them? Hope they would help you tell the others what you needed until you could speak the language? Now how would you feel if you were trying to tell this person you needed a drink, and they showed you where the bathroom was because they didn't understand you. So you asked again in the only language you knew, and then that person left you alone. What would that teach you? Would you trust that person? Would you think you were spoiled if that person stayed by you and tried to help you and make you feel safe?" I saw a light go on in his eyes.

—Barb Otterson, IBCLC; Spooner, WI

* Regarding the concept of when mothers offer the first breast first until done and then offer the other, it's okay if baby doesn't want it that time. Sometimes you feel like having desert after a meal, and sometimes you don't.

—Gail S. Hertz, MD, IBCLC; York, PA

* An analogy for the concept of "Don't wait until your baby cries to feed him." Imagine going to your favorite restaurant, being seated ready for your meal, and the waitress doesn't come to take your order. At first you're just irritated; more time passes, and you're pretty darn angry; and when your food does finally come, you're too upset to enjoy it.

—Gail S. Hertz, MD, IBCLC; York, PA

* An analogy to explain foremilk versus hindmilk is that hindmilk is higher in fat content than foremilk and is sort of like having cheesecake at the end of your meal. It leaves you feeling full and satisfied.

—Gail S. Hertz, MD, IBCLC; York, PA

* Try this one to explain the look of a baby when it's ready to eat versus the look when it's full after eating. At the beginning of the meal, the baby will have an intense look like when a little kid is going to open his birthday presents. At the end of the meal is that look that the family gets after eating Thanksgiving dinner. (I act this one out.)

—Gail S. Hertz, MD, IBCLC; York, PA

* An analogy for the dads: Babies' two favorite things to look at are faces and bullseyes. (I pause for effect as they ponder the bullseye part.) Think about what a breast looks like. They all "light up" when they make the connection.

—Gail S. Hertz, MD, IBCLC; York, PA

- Feeding is like a plumbing system. The baby feeding at the breast is what turns on the tap. We all have different types of plumbing, and for some people the milk may splutter out slowly to begin with, and for others it may gush out, almost faster than we want it. In time, as you and the baby get used to how your plumbing works, you will learn how to turn the tap on just as you want it or how to handle the type of plumbing you have. If the baby isn't positioned on properly, it's like he is trying to turn on the tap with a pair of boxing gloves. The tap may turn a little, just enough to get a little out, but its a long, hard job to get enough out to satisfy him. There's always milk there, just as there is always water when you turn on the tap. Although what is in the storage tank may be used, there is always more available from the mains. You are the well from which your baby drinks, and to keep your supply of drinkable quality you have to think about what you are putting into that well.

  —Jenny Lesley, NCT Counsellor; Worthing, England

- To say clearly and graphically what happens when areolar tissue is pinched and lifted toward the baby (usually to be stuffed into its half-closed mouth): Getting a corner of the pillowcase with no pillow! (Kathleen Bruce told me this one, and I think someone else gave it to her, maybe Diane Wiessinger.)

  —Rachel Myr, RN, RM; Kristiansand, Norway

- I'll disclose the way I let mothers know my attitude to painful feedings. I say pain is a sign that something is wrong, and that breastfeeding is supposed to resemble how we make babies rather than giving birth to them. You don't have to give birth very often; breastfeeding is supposed to be so comfortable that you want to do it many times every day, for months or years on end. (When I think about it, the frequency pattern for breastfeeding couples does bear some resemblance to the newly smitten-in-love—obsessed at first and then later able to do it while one partner eats, sleeps, reads a magazine, plays, or talks on the phone. Important disclaimer: Know your audience *well* before attempting to include this in teaching.)

  —Rachel Myr, RN, RM; Kristiansand, Norway

- The common question I am asked is "how do you burp your baby after a feed?" I generally say to the mums that it is always worth giving the baby a chance to bring up any wind they have, just by sitting them upright after they have fed, but not to dwell on it for too long. At that point, most of them start patting the baby on the back in an effort to work the wind up and ask "Is that right?" A few years ago I read a comical point of view in a parenting book, and I apologize for not being able to give a reference. It went along the lines of: Just imagine that you have been to a really lovely restaurant, and the atmosphere and company is magical. You have eaten some wonderful food, and now the meal is finished, and the waiter is coming out with the coffee and mints. The question is how would you feel if the waiter started banging you on the back to bring up your wind! I usually get a laugh and a nod from them.

  —Sally Elmes, RN, RM, IBCLC; Penrith, Australia

* Breastfeeding is like swimming. It's natural and instinctive in most animals, but people have to learn how. Breastfeeding is like dancing. The two partners each have to learn the steps. Even if one person knows how, if the other one doesn't, toes will get stepped on for a while.

  —Cynthia D. Payne, IBCLC; Williamstown, MA

* I, too, use the broccoli, driving, and healthy-eating-for-adults metaphors. Also dancing or love-making—adults don't always do either well to begin with—work well with a multipara who can't understand why this baby is harder to feed than the last! Comparisons to a new dancing partner, one who is less experienced than you, also work. Also, like Regina, I use the dinner idea—except I say doughnut—in NZ our doughnuts are big fat things, filled with cream and jam—and omelette. One won't fill you up for as long, but which is better for you?

  —Fiona Hermann, RN, RM, IBCLC; Hamilton, New Zealand

* I suggest "the little green men from Mars" approach. I also use this with my five-year-old when she's insistent about something but way off base. *The Little Green Men From Mars Approach*: You are the greeter/informant from the earth. The person with the irrational comments about breastfeeding practices is a little green man from Mars. The little green man from Mars (hereafter known as *lgmfm*) just sounds irrational because, of course, Mars is very different from Earth, and Martian laws don't apply. Now, if you need to explain something to a *lgmfm* that just arrived, you would break it down into simple parts, explain without being rude or patronizing, and be very matter of fact and very positive about the whole deal. Maybe it's not understood the first time. But, like the earthly law of gravity, just because the *lgmfm* doesn't understand it or agree with it, doesn't mean it's going to change to suit his needs or perceptions. Just be open and pleasant. If the *lgmfm* begins to get on your nerves, picture the bald green head and pointy ears that *lgmfm* have and keep smiling. Remember, you don't argue with a *lgmfm*—you educate. (If the *lgmfm* is looking for a fight, he'll have to try a different planet, thank you.)

  —Gail Hertz, MD, IBCLC; York, PA

* Nipple confusion or preference is controversial at our hospital. I explain to parents that newborns are learning to nurse and that they must suck differently on the breast and on a bottle. Switching back and forth can cause them confusion. I compare it to a person learning two foreign languages at the same time. They may say some words in French when they meant to speak Spanish.

  —Judy Hatfield, RNC, CCE, IBCLC; New Hartford, NY

* For a class or group, always feed the mamas. There's something about a snack that makes coming and chatting a bit more interesting. I think adults like to talk over food.

  —Pierrette Mimi Poinsett, MD, FAAP; Modesto, CA

- To discuss good latch-on and its importance in preventing sore nipples, I take an old sneaker with laces to class. I use the shoe to show how the nipple should fit in the baby's mouth. Everyone can relate to how sore and blistered a foot (nipple) would get if the tongue of the shoe were not pulled out all the way. The foot (nipple) would also get sore if one of the sides of the shoe (baby's lips) is rolled in. Also, how well can we walk if our foot is not in the shoe all the way (good milk transfer)?

  —Amy E. Uecker, BS, IBCLC; Mason, OH

- I have used the INFACT picture posters with great success in outlining the first half of my breastfeeding class in which the emphasis is on the importance of breastmilk, the frustrations of succeeding at breastfeeding in a community/society where it is not always valued, and sharing how breastmilk and breastfeeding complete a baby and initiate attachment behavior in the mother. Showing the approximately 8–10 posters with the accompanying blurbs addresses health issues, cost issues, and modesty issues that many parents are concerned about, gives me a visual springboard for discussions about "look at that baby," which helps the parents focus in on the baby part, the person part of breastfeeding, not just the "I should because I should" aspect of choice making.

  —Karen Foard, IBCLC; State College, PA

- During the first weeks postpartum, to help parents remember early feeding cues, suggest that they watch for squirming, stretching and squeaking *and* sucking, smacking and searching. Many people remember words best in groups of three. When saying these early cues, pause briefly between the two groups of three. This piques audience interest and curiosity about what you may say next. The grouping of all "S" words also facilitates retention and recall of these early feeding cues.

  —Deborah Tobin RN, BSN, IBCLC, LCCE; Springfield, VA

- I have been working with a family with many reservations about why they should continue to try to get their baby to breastfeed. They know the intellectual reasons but are bombarded with nice people's concerns for their own well-being. ("Why are you working so hard? Bottles and/or formula isn't so bad. Give yourself a break. You are torturing your baby.") First I explain that breastfeeding is the normal way a human baby should feed, that a baby who cannot breastfeed well, does not have a breastfeeding problem, but a feeding problem. (Whatever is causing the baby to do poorly at the breast remains in place with the bottle and often never gets addressed; We often see the baby struggling to take that uncontrolled bottle flow and the host of other problems that come when the bottle contains formula.) Like any physical or developmental challenge, breastfeeding often benefits from continued work on it as time passes and healthy growth, especially on pumped mom's milk is provided. Although our society does not yet see it as such, people who suggest giving up and switching to bottles of formula are saying nothing different than someone who says to a mother whose year-old baby does not yet walk, "Well don't work with him on that, just put him in leg braces to make it easy for him, and that will be good enough." Most babies, if the mother protects her supply and keeps working and expecting the baby to catch on, will do exactly that. Bottles and braces can be useful as tools, but the goal is to do the thing the body should and that most can in time. I find that this lack of understanding about breastfeeding as normal and as something that is necessary to work toward is still very foreign to most people. I hope it helps the mother, who is working so hard for her baby, to feel there is a damn good reason to do so.)

—Judy LeVan Fram, IBCLC; Brooklyn, NY

* One position at breast is success. More is just variety. Just like with lovemaking.

—Linda J. Smith, BSE, FACCE, IBCLC; Dayton, OH

FORK IT OVER

GOAL

To understand eating ability and patterns with different feeding devices and different conditions

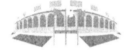

BEST AUDIENCE

Any

TIME REQUIRED

10 minutes

HOW TO PLAY

Gather several eating utensils: fork, spoon, table knife, chopsticks, tweezers, cheap plastic fork, small cup, dropper, very large drinking tumbler or glass, straws, baby bottle with teat (nipple), salad tongs, etc.

Tell the group that they are going on a cosmic journey to many places all around the universe, which have different eating customs. They will have to learn to use different utensils and devices, possibly eat or drink unusual products, and cope with foods or travel conditions that may affect their alertness and coordination.

Encourage a free-wheeling discussion of the experiences that might occur when using each of the utensils for the first time.

    a. Would it be easy to use chopsticks after mastering using salad tongs?

    b. How could you eat with tweezers after drinking a beverage that affected concentration?

    c. Does drinking cup size affect how you consume liquids?

Correlate this to infants' experiences with alternate feeding devices, birth medications, changing composition of mother's milk, learning to eat solid (family) foods, and switching between breast and bottle/teat.

How To Make
Breastfeeding Difficult

....

GOAL

To identify barriers and common myths that interfere with breastfeeding. This game uses reverse psychology, because getting bad advice is often worse than getting no advice at all.

BEST AUDIENCE

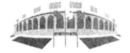

All

TIME REQUIRED

10–15 minutes

HOW TO PLAY

Using a chalkboard, blank overhead transparency, or flip chart pad, ask the group to name everything they can think of that would make breastfeeding more difficult for a mother. Write down the answers.

Afterward, discuss why these barriers and myths persist. Some people in the audience will be surprised to find out that some of the "rules" they have learned are actually counterproductive to breastfeeding.

Compare the new collection to my list. I use my list as a handout to new parents, warning them, "If someone tries to tell you anything that's on this list, or does anything on this list, then know they are not helping you breastfeed. This is a list of what *not* to do." I also hand out my list to professionals, threatening that if they do anything on the list to parents, I will come and haunt them forever.

154

HOW TO MAKE BREASTFEEDING DIFFICULT[2]

1. Tell the mother to "feed on a four-hour schedule" or "get the baby on a schedule." This results in a low milk supply and a hungry, frustrated baby and frustrated parents. Be sure to blame the crying on breastfeeding.

2. Be sure to "get the baby used to a bottle." This can result in a confused baby who refuses the breast. It's also a great way to lower the milk supply and undermine the mother's confidence.

3. Tell her she doesn't have enough milk if

   "The baby wants to nurse again after only two to three hours."

   "The baby will take two ounces of formula after nursing."

   "Your breasts aren't full and uncomfortable all the time."

   Because milk supply insecurity is the primary cause of lactation failure, this will introduce an element of doubt and fear to the whole process.

4. Tell her she can't or shouldn't nurse if

   "She wants to eat chocolate (or Mexican food or cabbage, etc.)."

   "She smokes or wants to take medication."

   "She's going back to work/school in a few weeks."

   "She wants to go out in public; nursing requires privacy."

   "Her breasts are too small (or large)."

   "Her mother couldn't."

   "She's too nervous." . . . etc., etc., etc.

   Find as many reasons for *not* breastfeeding as you can and look for *any* reason to interrupt it. Put as much distance between mother and baby as possible.

5. "Dad should give the baby a bottle or he'll feel left out." This is another good way to minimize the importance of breastfeeding.

continues

continued

6. Tell her it may hurt to breastfeed and that sore, cracked nipples are normal. Pain is an excellent adverse stimulus. Don't teach her how to position the baby correctly. Do give her a nipple shield, give the baby lots of bottles to disrupt the proper suck, and tell her to rub her nipples with a rough towel to "condition" them.

7. Tell her to give the baby formula, glucose water, and cereal right from the beginning to "make the baby sleep." This is another good way to ensure inadequate milk supply.

8. Tell her that her milk might be too rich or too thin. This will further shatter her confidence. And, be sure to tell her every "horror story" you've ever heard about breastfeeding.

9. Separate her from her baby at birth and show by your actions that water, formula, pacifiers, and scheduled feedings are the appropriate way to care for the baby. Because she is especially vulnerable at this time and will follow your example, be sure to tell her how little breastfeeding matters.

10. Don't teach her the normal course of infant behavior. Don't warn her about growth spurts and frequency days. Don't call or visit her, and be sure to leave her alone in the critical first two weeks.

11. Give her plenty of formula samples to take home to further weaken her confidence. Make sure that the literature you give her has many references to formula and doesn't tell her how to maintain her milk supply.

All these tactics, individually and collectively, will discourage breastfeeding.

[2] © Linda J. Smith, 1986, 1998.

MAKING MILK

GOAL

To understand and apply the principles/physiology of milk synthesis

BEST AUDIENCE

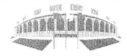

Any; these analogies help parents and professionals.

TIME REQUIRED

A few minutes each

HOW TO PLAY

The old familiar concept of "supply meets demand" still applies to breastfeeding. However, new research shows that breast storage capacity has an important role in establishing and maintaining milk supply. The secretory cells in the alveoli generate milk at the highest rate when the lumen is the emptiest. As the lumen fills with milk, the secretion rate drops.

The following page contains analogies to help understand this concept.

ICE MAKER ANALOGY

An automatic icemaker in a refrigerator generates ice wedges or cubes, which drop into a basket or deep tray. A mechanical arm is positioned over the basket, so that as the amount of ice in the basket increases, the arm raises up and slows down the flow of water into the freezing unit, which reduces the rate at which more cubes are made. When the basket is full, the arm is at its highest point and completely shuts off the flow of water to the freezing compartment. No more ice is made until the basket is emptied and the arm releases the flow of water again.

This illustrates the principle that removing milk triggers the cells to make more milk.

TOILET TANK ANALOGY

A toilet tank holds only a certain volume of water. When the toilet is flushed, the water drains out rapidly and then the drain is sealed again. The water intake valve opens, and more water flows rapidly into the tank to fill it. A floating ball on a control arm connects to the water inlet valve. As the tank fills, the floating ball rises, causing the inflow of water to slow down and finally to stop. More water does not flow into the tank until the next time the tank is flushed.

The number of flushings per day determines the total volume of water used by the system. If it is flushed 10 times, more water will have flowed through than if it was flushed five times. The size of the tank did not change, but the volume of water cycling in the system was twice as much.

This illustrates that more frequent feeds = increased volume of milk generated per day, even though the amount of milk obtained in any single feed or pumping session remains the same.

Clinical implication and warning: Do not assume that any and all babies are actually removing milk when they are at breast. A baby with a poor suck will leave most of the milk in the breast, triggering early involution. The solution is to observe babies very carefully, and if there is doubt of the baby's ability to effectively get milk from the breast, encourage the mother to *also* use another method of milk removal (hand expression or pumping), and continue to follow the dyad closely.

MILK FAT PROPERTIES[3]

GOAL

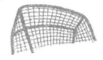

To understand variations in fat levels in milk, color of milk, and other aspects of milk

BEST AUDIENCE

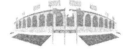

Any. These analogies help parents and professionals alike.

TIME REQUIRED

A few minutes to collect samples and observe

HOW TO PLAY

Materials needed:

* Test-tube rack and about 12 tubes with stoppers. Tubes used for drawing blood can be used or any similar tube with capacity of about 10–30 cc.

* One or two breastfeeding mothers willing to express some milk

* Labels for the tubes

Ask the mothers to give small samples of milk (about 10 cc) collected from each breast in the following manners:

* Mother A, right breast, just prior to a feed or with a full breast

* Mother A, right breast, just after a feed or at the end of a pumping session

---

[3] **Source:** Peter Hartmann, PhD; University of Western Australia in Perth. I saw Dr. Hartmann do this exercise/demonstration at a conference in Orlando, FL, in 1995 or 1996.

- Mother A, left breast, same two samples as preceding

- Mother B, same four samples as preceding.

Arrange the tubes in the rack so that the labels are visible. Have students view the tubes either by walking to where the rack is displayed, or pass around the rack with the tubes in place, being careful not to shake or disturb the tubes.

After a few minutes, the milk will start to separate, and fat will rise to the top. Make the following observations, especially noting differences in the fat layer:

- Any one breast, pre- and post-feed

- Both breasts of one mother, both pre-feed and post-feed

- Differences in pre-feed samples from both breasts and both mothers

- Differences in post-feed samples from both breasts and both mothers

- Color(s) of fat layers

- Color(s) of other layers

Gently swirl one of the tubes to show how easily milk fat rehomogenizes back into solution. Let the samples stand for several hours or overnight. Repeat the observations and comparisons.

If possible, compare the samples a few days later. Even without refrigeration, there may not be obvious spoilage of the milk.

When finished, discard all milk samples and clean the tubes thoroughly. Sterilize the tubes before the next use by boiling, autoclaving, or another method.

MULTITASKING MAMA[4]

GOAL

To simulate the effect of the chaotic environment of the new mother who has multiple competing demands on her ability to learn or listen to instruction.

BEST AUDIENCE

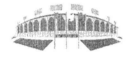

Any. This game is especially effective with professional audiences.

TIME REQUIRED

10–15 minutes

HOW TO PLAY

Prepare the stage with an inflatable mallet, pad of self-adhesive notes, a pen, sturdy table, and three chairs. If you can't find an inflatable mallet, use a small pillow, wrapping paper tube core, soft foam "noodle" or other harmless weapon. Put one chair on top of the sturdy table and one chair on each side of the table. All chairs should face the group.

Ask for three volunteers who are wearing shoes with laces.

* One volunteer will be the *mother*. She sits in the chair on top of the table. Her shoes will be accessible by the instructor.

* A second will be the *baby*, who is unhappy and will cry non-stop for a few minutes. This volunteer will sit in one of the side chairs.

---

[4]**Source:** Carol Schlef, RNC, MSW, IBCLC. Carol presented this hilarious role-play at a conference in Florida in January, 2000, and I loved it.

* The *stressor*, who sits in the other chair, will wield the mallet and use the self-adhesive notes. The notes represent the stresses that a mother faces in the first few days post birth. Ask the class, "What are these stresses?" Audience will supply many common ones: lack of sleep, fatigue, sore bottom, sore breasts, too many visitors, laundry, meal preparation, other children, etc. Write one stressor on each sticky note and stick them to the table under the chair. Continue until there are more than a few notes prepared.

To begin the instructor plays the nurse or LC who is going to teach the *mother* how to tie her shoes in a new way.

* The LC faces the *mother* and begins to teach her the new skill by demonstrating on the mother's own shoes, explaining while she works. The mother tries to lean forward to see what's going on.

* Just as the LC begins her demonstration, the *baby* begins to cry and continues for the duration of the demonstration.

* Simultaneously, the *stressor* starts bopping the *mother* with the mallet and places a stress note somewhere on her body. This continues until all the notes are placed all over the mother.

* The LC continues with her instruction, oblivious to the *mother*, *baby*, and *stressor's* reactions to all of this.

* When the shoelace-tying demonstration is done, stop the activity.

Discussion—invite feedback and comments from the group:

* How does this translate to new mothers and breastfeeding instruction?

* What was it like for the baby in this scenario? For the mother? For the instructor?

* Is it reasonable that the mother could even *begin* to learn a new skill, given everything that is going on?

* What can we do to improve this situation for the mother and baby?

RULES OF THE GAME[5]

GOAL

To succinctly state "rules" for breastfeeding, which are the core principles for success

BEST AUDIENCE

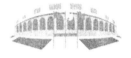

Any. These can also be used as posters.

TIME REQUIRED

A few minutes

HOW TO PLAY

COACH SMITH'S RULES

Rule #1: Feed the baby.

Rule #2: The mother is right.

Rule #3: It's her baby.

Rule #4: Nobody knows everything.

Rule #5: There's another way.

[5] **Source:** I first heard the phrase "Rule #1 is Feed the Baby" from Trina Vosti and Andrea Van Outryve, who were presenting a talk at the 1998 ILCA conference.

KAREN GROMADA'S RULES

Rule #1: Feed the baby.

Rule #2: Move the milk.

Rule #3: Keep the breastfeeding couple together.

—Karen Kerkhoff Gromada, RN, MSN, IBCLC; Cincinnati, OH

CHRIS MULFORD'S VARIATION

Rule #1: Keep the dyad together, which will result in . . .

Rule #2: Feed the baby; and

Rule #3: Move the milk.

—Chris Mulford, BA, RN, IBCLC; Swarthmore, PA

TRIPLE PLAY

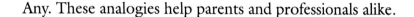

GOAL

To understand the special nature of the mother-baby dyad

BEST AUDIENCE

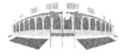

Any. These analogies help parents and professionals alike.

TIME REQUIRED

Variable

HOW TO PLAY

The mother-baby dyad is unique in nature. Both people have physical and emotional needs and aspects; yet each is dependent and interdependent on the other. Trying to understand human lactation without considering the *baby* is futile; trying to understand the breastfed baby outside of the context of the *mother* is equally inappropriate. The *dyad* is more than the sum of its parts. The mother and her milk supply is one aspect; the baby and his ability to obtain milk is another; and their unique biophysical relationship is the third.

UNICEF and WHO discuss breastfeeding in the context of promotion, support, and protection. Promotion is the "why," and includes motivation to begin, counseling skills, and the concept that "milk is good." Protection refers to the context and circumstances in which breastfeeding takes place—the "where"—and includes facilities to breastfeed, public acceptance, and the concept that "It's good to breastfeed." Support provides the foundation and is the "how" aspect. Support includes management skills of milk supply, comfort, and problem solving, and the concept that "I can make milk."

The following page contains ways to illustrate the three-in-one nature of breastfeeding or breastfeeding care.

TRIANGLE IMAGE

I place *support* at the base/foundation of the triangle because if the mother doesn't know how to make enough milk, or it hurts her to breastfeed, the other aspects (promotion and protection) won't matter for long. I also place the dyad *relationship* at the base/foundation position because understanding the interrelated and interconnected physiology of breastfeeding is fundamental to understanding either maternal anatomy and physiology or infant development.

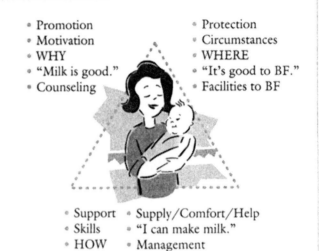

- Promotion
- Motivation
- WHY
- "Milk is good."
- Counseling

- Protection
- Circumstances
- WHERE
- "It's good to BF."
- Facilities to BF

- Support
- Skills
- HOW

- Supply/Comfort/Help
- "I can make milk."
- Management

BRAIDED CORD

This idea originated with the Nursing Mothers group in Philadelphia, PA, and was described to me by Nikki Lee, RN, MSN, IBCLC.

I bought thick satiny drapery cord in red, blue, and gold and bound the cut ends with thread. Then I braided the three strands together. Any one strand is unique, and together the braid is exceptionally strong. A flaw in any one strand may affect the other two, as well as the assembled braid.

THREE-LEGGED STOOL

This was first described by Kathleen Auerbach, PhD, IBCLC in "Breastfeeding Promotion: Why It Doesn't Work." *J Hum Lact* 1990, 6(2): 45. Kathy eloquently describes how any one "leg," support alone, protection alone, or promotion alone, will not be sufficient to establish breastfeeding as the cultural norm. All three aspects must be in place simultaneously, just as a stool must have all three legs to support the load.

Martha Grodrian, RD, LD, IBCLC had a local carpenter build a wooden three-legged stool, with the legs fitted slightly loosely so that she could demonstrate the concepts.

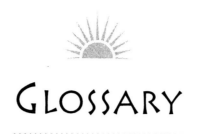

GLOSSARY

AAP American Academy of Pediatrics

APGAR score Ten-point assessment of newborns done at one and five minutes postbirth.

The Baby Friendly Hospital Initiative™; Baby Friendly Hospital™ Designations awarded by UNICEF to hospitals and birth facilities that implement the *Ten Steps to Successful Breastfeeding* as defined by UNICEF and the World Health Organization.

CNS Central nervous system

Colostrum Secretion of the mammary gland during pregnancy and early postbirth

D&C Dilation and curettage, a procedure to dilate the cervical canal of the uterus so that the surface lining of the uterus can be scraped

FACCE Fellow, American College of Childbirth Education

Family bed Situation in which a baby is sleeping with his or her parents in the same bed

Football hold Baby is held semi-vertically at breast, with the legs tucked under the mother's arm

Gaffer's tape Duct tape or other sturdy adhesive tape used to secure cords to the floor or carpeting in meeting rooms

Hindmilk Milk that flows late in an individual breastfeed. Hindmilk is higher in fat than foremilk (milk that flows early in an individual feed).

IBCLC International Board Certified Lactation Consultant, a person who has passed the international credentialing exam administered by the International Board of Lactation Consultant Examiners (IBLCE)

IBLCE International Board of Lactation Consultant Examiners

ILCA   International Lactation Consultant Association

Innocenti Declaration   The Innocenti Declaration on the Protection, Promotion and Support of Breastfeeding, issued in August 1990 by 30 governments meeting in Florence, Italy; sets four important global operational targets: "All Governments should have: appointed a national breastfeeding coordinator of appropriate authority, and established a multisectoral breastfeeding committee composed of representatives from relevant government departments, non-governmental organizations, and health professional associations; ensured that every facility providing maternity services practices all ten of the Ten Steps to Successful Breastfeeding; taken action to give effect to the principles and aim of all Articles of the International Code and subsequent relevant World Health Assembly Resolutions in their entirety; enacted imaginative legislation protecting the breastfeeding rights of working women and established means for its enforcement."

Intestinal colonization   At birth, the infant's gastrointestinal tract is sterile. Human milk helps establish growth of normal (non-harmful) bacteria in the gut.

Kangaroo Care   A program of skin-to-skin contact between parent and child, which is especially beneficial for premature babies

Lactalbumin   A soluble protein found in milk

Lactational Amennorrhea Method (LAM)   A natural family planning method based on exclusive breastfeeding: if the baby is less than six months old, the mother is exclusively breastfeeding, and menstruation has not resumed, the chance of an unplanned pregnancy is less than two percent.

Let-down reflex   *See* Milk ejection reflex (MER)

LLL Leader   Volunteer mother-support group leader accredited by La Leche League International

Madonna hold   Also known as the cradle position. The mother holds her baby with the baby's head in the crook of her elbow and the legs extended across her body.

Mature milk   Milk produced from two weeks postbirth onward

Meconium   First stool of a newborn baby. Meconium is thick, dark green or black and tarry.

Milk ejection reflex (MER)   Rapid flow of milk due to the action of the posterior pituitary hormone oxytocin contracting the myoepithelial cells in the mammary alveoli. Oxytocin is released in response to the infant's sucking at breast.

"Neo-Mull-Soy" and "Cho-Free"   Infant formulas that lacked chloride, manufactured by Syntex Laboratories in the late 1970's

NICU   Newborn Intensive Care Unit (intensive care nursery)

Positioning and latch-on techniques   Various positions and movements to hold the baby and help him or her begin breastfeeding

Regression milk   Milk produced during weaning

Rooming-in   The practice of keeping a new mother and her newborn in the same hospital room

SigA   Secretory Immunoglobulin A.

Subjects and controls   In a research study using an experimental design, the subjects receive the intervention, while the controls do not.

Transitional milk   Milk produced on days two through fourteen postbirth

UNICEF   United Nations Children's Fund

VBAC   Vaginal Birth after Cesarean

WHO   World Health Organization

WHO Code   The WHO/UNICEF *International Code of Marketing of Breastmilk Substitutes* was adopted by a Resolution (WHA34.22) of the World Health Assembly in 1981. The International Code bans all promotion of bottle-feeding and sets out requirements for labeling and information on infant feeding. Any activity that undermines breastfeeding also violates the aim and spirit of the Code. The Code and its subsequent World Health Assembly Resolutions are intended as a minimum requirement in all countries.

BIBLIOGRAPHY

ASPO/Lamaze. *Teacher Certification Program*. Washington DC: ASPO/Lamaze, 1981.

Auerbach KG. Beyond the issue of accuracy: evaluating patient education materials for breastfeeding mothers. *J Hum Lact* 1988; 4: 108–110.

Cadwell K, Arnold LDW, Turner-Maffei C, and Smith LJ (eds). *The Curriculum in Support of the Ten Steps to Successful Breastfeeding: An 18 Hour Interdisciplinary Breastfeeding Management Course for the United States*. Washington, DC: United States Dept. of Health and Human Services, 1999. Order #98-0264.

Childbirth Graphics, a division of WRS Group, Ltd. PO Box 21207, Waco, TX 76702-1207, phone 800-299-3366, ext. 287, fax 888-977-7653, www.childbirthgraphics.com.

Hale T, *Medications and Mothers' Milk*, Amarillo, Texas: Pharmasoft Publishing Company, 2000.

Hilbers S. San Antonio, TX: Childbirth Education Workshop, 1988

International Childbirth Education Association. *Teacher Certification Program*. Minneapolis MN: International Childbirth Education Association, 1983.

Jones E. *Teaching Adults: An Active Learning Approach*. Washington, DC: National Association for the Education of Young Children, 1986.

Knowles M. *The Adult Learner: A Neglected Species*. Houston, TX: Gulf Publishing Co, 1973.

La Leche League International. *Human Relations Workbook*. Schaumburg, IL: La Leche League International, 1982.

Lactnet. http://peach.ease.lsoft.com/archives/lactnet.html.

Lawrence RA, Lawrence RM. *Breastfeeding, a Guide for the Medical Profession*, 5th edition. St. Louis: Mosby, 1999.

Lowe D. *PowerPoint© for Windows 95© for Dummies©*. Foster City, CA: IDG Books, 1995.

Mager R. *Preparing Instructional Objectives, Third edition*. Atlanta, GA: The Center for Effective Performance, 1997.

McIntyre E. Breastfeeding management: helping the mother help herself. *Breastfeeding Review* 1991; July: 129–32.

Palmer G. *The Politics of Breastfeeding*. London: Pandora Press, 1988; revised 1993.

Rabb MY. *The Presentation Design Book*. Chapel Hill, NC: Ventana Press, 1993.

Riordan J. Readable, relevant, and reliable: the three R's of breastfeeding pamphlets. *Breastfeeding Abstracts* 1985; 5: 5–6.

UNICEF. *Facts for Life: A Communication Challenge*. New York: UNICEF; 1991: 15–21.

Wiessinger D. A breastfeeding teaching tool using a sandwich analogy for latch-on. *J Hum Lact* 1998; 14(1): 51–56.

Williams LV. *Teaching for the Two-Sided Mind*. New York: Simon and Schuster, 1983.

Lightning Source UK Ltd.
Milton Keynes UK
UKOW02f1207280813

216046UK00009BA/39/P